Understanding
Man's Search for Meaning

Other books by Elisabeth Lukas

Meaning and Suffering

The Therapist and the Soul

In the series
Viktor Frankl's Living Logotherapy:

Understanding *Man's Search for Meaning*:
Reflections on Viktor Frankl's Logotherapy

A Unique Approach to Family Counseling:
Logotherapy, Crisis, and Youth

Stillness and Concentration:
Logotherapy Applied to Tinnitus and Chronic Illness

Meaningful Living:
Introduction to Logotherapy Theory and Practice

Understanding *Man's Search for Meaning:*

Reflections on Viktor Frankl's Logotherapy

Elisabeth Lukas

Translated by
Joseph Fabry, Howard Smith, Bianca Hirsch, & James O'Meara
Edited by Charles McLafferty, Jr.

Book 1: *Viktor Frankl's Living Logotherapy* series

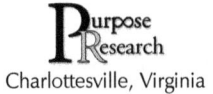
Charlottesville, Virginia

© 2020, 1981-2020 by The Elisabeth Lukas Archive. All international rights reserved
Published with the kind permission of Profil Verlag, Munich, except as noted below.

No part of this book may be reproduced by any mechanical, photographic, or electronic process, or in the form of a recording, nor may it be stored in a retrieval system, transmitted, or otherwise copied for public or private use—other than for fair use—without the written permission of the publisher. All quotes are believed to be fair use.

Published by Purpose Research, Box 5032, Charlottesville, Virginia 22905 USA
http://PurposeResearch.com   charles@purposeresearch.com
Back cover photograph © 2014 Charles McLafferty, Jr.
Cover design, layout, and typesetting by Purpose Research

These manuscripts were originally translated by Joseph B. Fabry, Howard T. Smith, Bianca Zwang-Hirsch, and James O'Meara, whose service to the next generation of logotherapists is deeply appreciated.

The following chapters (translated by Joseph Fabry) are reprinted gratefully from *The International Forum for Logotherapy*: 1: "The logotherapeutic view of human nature"; 2: "Logotherapy: Health through meaning"; 7: "Correcting the image"; 8: "On Overcoming the tragic triad."

The following chapters were keynote addresses to World Congresses of Logotherapy, privately published by the author: 3: "What is special about logotherapy?" (1995, Toronto); 4: "Survival—To what end?" (1983, Regensburg, Germany); 5: "Waiting for Godot? The logotherapeutic alternative" (1993, Toronto); 9: "'Key Words' as a guarantee against the imposition of values" and 10: "A person's admission into self-responsibility" (1982, Hartford, Connecticut).

Chapter 6: "From self-actualization to global responsibility" was originally published in *The road to self-esteem and social conscience: The proceedings of the Seventh World Congress of Logotherapy* (1989, Finck, W., Finck, M. & Larson, L, eds.). Berkeley: Institute of Logotherapy Press.

Chapter 11: "Reflections on the future (2014)" is reprinted with permission of Springer Nature (Switzerland) from *Logotherapy and Existential Analysis: Proceedings of the Viktor Frankl Institute Vienna*, (2016, Batthyany, A., ed.). The speech was originally published in: Lukas, E. (2015). *Das Schicksal waltet - der Mensch gestaltet - mit Versöhnung und Frieden* (3rd ed.). Perchtoldsdorf: Plattform Martikenek Verlag and the translation is also reprinted with permission of Plattform Martikenek Verlag.

Poems after each chapter are from Lukas, E. (1992). *Meaningful lines: Logophilosophical wisdom* (Hirsch, B. & Fabry, J., trans.). Berkeley: Institute of Logotherapy Press.

This book is published for educational purposes only and is not intended for the diagnosis and/or treatment of medical or mental health disorders. Readers who need help with any such disorder are encouraged to consult with a logotherapist or other qualified professional

For more information about the work of Elisabeth Lukas around the world, please visit the Lukas Archives: http://elisabeth-lukas-archiv.de

For more information about training in logotherapy and existential analysis search for "Viktor Frankl Institute" and "Elisabeth Lukas Archive" on the web.

ISBN: 978-1-948523-20-2 (Hardcover)
978-1-948523-00-4 (Paperback)

Library of Congress Control Number: 2019951172

9 8 7 6 5 4 3 2 1

Contents

Foreword vii

1. The Logotherapeutic View of Human Nature 1
2. Logotherapy: Health Through Meaning 7
3. What is Special About Logotherapy? 21
4. Survival—To What End? Answers to Questions of Fate 37
5. Waiting for Godot? The Logotherapeutic Alternative 51
6. From Self-Actualization to Global Responsibility 71
7. Correcting the Image 89
8. On Overcoming the Tragic Triad: Suffering, Guilt, and Death . 95
9. "Key words" as a Guarantee Against the Imposition of Values . 107
10. A Person's Admission Into Self-Responsibility: Reducing the Relapse Rate in Psychotherapy 117
11. Reflections on our Future (2014) 135

Foreword

I met Elisabeth Lukas in 1993 at the World Congress of Logotherapy in Toronto. It was my first World Congress, and I had completed the Introduction to Logotherapy course the day before. It was a flashbulb moment for me, and years later I wrote:

> The auditorium where she was to speak was packed, and I sat in the front row of the balcony. She was introduced warmly, if not effusively, and received an award from one of Canada's Ministers of Parliament.
>
> The topic was "Waiting for Godot: A logotherapeutic alternative." I was skeptical that Beckett's play of despair and futility could be connected to the hopeful message of Frankl's logotherapy. Gerhard, her husband, sat on the stage, next to the overhead projector, with a table full of transparencies. There was an air of anticipation as she walked to the podium and put on her reading glasses.
>
> Lukas began by talking about the path of life, and asked us to imagine ourselves walking through a wilderness. She spoke of our need for a signpost of direction, a "cloud of hope" like the Biblical cloud that led the Jews out of Egypt. She painted word pictures of a vision, a personal "cloud" of transcendence that belongs to us. Lukas then connected all of this to Beckett's play, to show how the characters ignored repeated opportunities to find meaning. They even noticed a single cloud passing by, a quickly forgotten chimera.
>
> She ended by pointing out that the first two acts of the play have finished, and the curtain is now rising on the third act, "the third millennium after Christ." We, humanity, are

the players in this new act of Godot. Will we, as a people, continue to bypass and ignore the call of meaning? Or will we seek, find, recognize, and respond to the persistent call of this cloud which appears before us?[1]

As will be seen in the pages of this volume (and throughout her writings), Elisabeth Lukas has developed and applied the insights and ideas of Viktor Frankl in new ways, applications that are unexpected, even surprising. The reader may even conclude that she has expanded Frankl's ideas into new arenas.

The experience that we have of the unexpected—the surprise with which we react to Lukas' insights—bring us to confront the unknown in our own lives and to discover new possibilities that are unanticipated. Just as Lukas opens new doors for her clients, so in our lives can we discover new doors that await us, as well as doors that beckon to those we endeavor to help.

One trademark of Lukas' teaching has been that, at the end of the course of training, Lukas challenges students with the responsibility they now have to find the unique meanings to which they are called. This was termed "living logotherapy" by Frankl, and Lukas has emphasized that it is not enough just to memorize the theory or to so learn the techniques that we can become exact practitioners. Frankl often pointed out that logotherapy is not a practice; it is an art.

Lukas (and Frankl) make us responsible for finding our own art of helping others. In so doing, they give us the keys to meaning and purpose. But this is merely knowledge until we activate it uniquely in our own lives… for ourselves and, above all, for others. Lukas assures us by her example: What an adventure awaits us—the world of meaning!

About this series

Over the years, Lukas has written more than 50 books, which have been translated into 19 languages. She has given keynote addresses and lectures

---

[1] McLafferty, C. L., Jr. (1997). *Spirituality in three theories of psychology: A qualitative study (Doctoral dissertation, University of Virginia).* (58), Dissertation Abstracts International, 58, 03b: 1567, pp. 94-95.
Note: The entire 1993 keynote address appears as Chapter 5 of this book.

at numerous universities and conferences, including many of the World Congresses of Logotherapy. Her writings have been translated into English for print in books and journals, particularly *The international forum for logotherapy: Journal of search for meaning*. For years, I have wanted to collect these writings in a book form. I am personally grateful for the support of Elisabeth Lukas the Lukas Archive, as well as many others who have given so unselflishly of their time and energy to help move this project forward.

This volume, *Understanding Man's Search for Meaning: Reflections on Viktor Frankl's logotherapy,* contains some of the most insightful and profound expansions of logotherapy into the problems of our time. Many of these chapters are drawn from keynote addresses to World Congresses of Logotherapy. Until now, most of the English versions have been privately published, though some have appeared in the *International forum for logotherapy.*

A second volume, *A unique approach to family counseling: Logotherapy, crisis, and youth,* focuses on the application of logotherapy in families and relationships. It includes articles from the *International forum*, book chapters, and keynote speeches.

The third book presents two lines of thought. The first part of the book is a translation of *Stillness and concentration: Logotherapy for tinnitus and chronic diseases.* The rest of the volume contains articles and presentations that fall broadly under the topic of "psychotherapy with dignity."

A new edition of *Meaningful living: Introduction to logotherapy theory and practice* is the fourth book in the series. Part A contains a revision of the 1984 classic, *Meaningful living: Logotherapeutic guide to health.* Part B adds an extended synopsis of logotherapy by Elisabeth Lukas and Bianca Hirsch originally published in the *Comprehensive handbook of psychotherapy, vol. 3.* Many of the cases summarized in the article can be found in more detail in the original text of *Meaningful living,* and are cross-referenced throughout. This archival article also documents the history of logotherapy as of 2002.

To the extent possible, these books have been edited for a new generation of logotherapists. For example, in 1984 when the original edition of

Meaningful Living was first printed, cassette players were in wide use—remember the Walkman? (Sony still makes a version of it, but cassettes are nearly extinct.) Sentences have been restructured whenever possible to use inclusive language (including sex, race, culture, and gender identity) and to avoid labeling (e.g., "person with an addiction disorder" instead of "addict") in accordance with the *Publication Manual of the American Psychological Association* (6th ed). Further, the translation of these concepts from German into English occasionally resulted in difficult-to-understand passages, and these have been revised and even rewritten. If, as a result of this work, meaning has been lost or changed, that is solely my fault, and for that I take full responsibility. Hopefully, the inherent meaning will shine through when English words are inadequate to express it.

It is hoped that these books will serve to kindle interest in the meaning possibilities available to all of us, and in so doing ignite the flames of meaning among those who sense there is something more to life than having possessions, money, a beautiful home, a prestigious position, and a multitude of friends. To those enduring long periods of unemployment during the Great Depression nearly a century ago, Frankl noted that the problem wasn't a lack of money, but a lack of meaning.

To each reader, no matter at what stage in life, regardless of your setbacks, failures, and fate, there awaits a purpose that only you can fulfill, one for which you were created. It is the discovery of, orientation to, and *action on* this possibility that brings meaning. Even a few minutes a day pursuing this unique life mission will result in a harvest of positive fruits and help you to build a monument of meaning that can never be taken away… in time or in eternity.

Charles McLafferty, Jr.
University of Virginia
June, 2019

CHAPTER 1

The Logotherapeutic View of Human Nature

The full picture of the human being is slowly emerging from the assumptions and discoveries of early psychology. Psychoanalysts perceived that human beings are shaped by their past experiences, including childhood traumas and conflicts. Behavior therapists recognized that individuals are also shaped by how they have been reinforced to behave.

Humanists and existentialists of the postwar years have pointed out that human beings are more than mere victims of their past or mere results of their learning; they are masters of their lives to a greater extent than they have been given credit for.

A therapist who sees patients primarily as "victims" and "results" will focus on what's wrong with them and neglect their capacity to develop what's right. In the early 1930s, Viktor Frankl was the first psychiatrist to point out that, in order to make and to keep patients healthy, medical professionals must not neglect the *human spirit* and its *defiant power* that can take a stand against past traumas and faulty learning, and thus release the self-healing power of the human being. He advocated the idea that therapists are more than interpreters or manipulators: they are people who take patients and their complaints at face value instead of assuming hidden motives and misguided learning.

OVERCOMING BASIC ASSUMPTIONS

A therapist has to overcome two basic, flawed, assumptions of earlier psychological theories about human nature. The first is the assumption that even adults are not accountable for their decisions—one might call this the assumption of an a priori guardianship. The second assumption is that human beings are exclusively oriented toward seeking pleasure and gaining advantages for themselves.

In psychoanalytical philosophy, the first assumption of a priori guardianship is expressed by presenting the unconscious, with its repressed drives and impulses, as a ready excuse for harmful behavior. For example, a murderer kills because of being overwhelmed by repressed aggressiveness rooted in a lack of love experienced in childhood. Behaviorists frame a murder as a result of the killer not having learned any other reaction to a provocation but to hit or to behave in an uncontrolled manner; the killer's aggressiveness has been reinforced, one way or another, and thus learned behavior patterns escalate, to include murder. Human beings are seen as preprogrammed automatons that can no longer control their actions. The a priori guardianship is thus explained by behaviorists in a different way than by psychoanalysts, but the result is the same—an excuse for irresponsible behavior.

The question is not raised as to whether a human being, even under conditions of extreme anger or excitement, may be able to retain at least some veneer of freedom to decide whether or not to kill. The question forces psychologists to deal with such unscientific and unquantifiable concepts as conscience, responsibility, and guilt. A positive answer would presuppose some degree of freedom of will, which neither orthodox psychoanalysis nor orthodox behaviorism is willing to grant. Freedom of will is not compatible with seeing the person as a driven creature or automaton shaped by forces of repression or reinforcements. Freedom of will opens a new dimension in which the old hypotheses of cause and effect are inadequate.

The second assumption—that the human being is motivated by the search for hedonic pleasure and material advantages—seemed justified by psychological research. Psychoanalysts portray human nature as striving for the satisfaction of drives and needs, and neurosis was a possible consequence

1. Logotherapeutic View of Human Nature

when this chase after pleasure was blocked. Behavior therapists tended to see human nature reacting to rewards and punishments, mostly material in nature. In both theoretical stances, human behavior is motivated by the continuing pursuit of pleasure, material success, and recognition.

Frankl's early warning—that the will to pleasure and the will to success, though important motivations, were secondary to *the will to meaning*—went unheard for a long time. Then affluence came to the post-World-War Western world, with its abundance of material goods, luxuries, shorter working hours, and the possibilities to enjoy pleasures reserved previously only to the idle rich.

Yet, contrary to psychological theories, such individuals were not healthier. The number of people prone to mental illness, violence, suicide, addiction, lack of direction, and sexual disorders increased sharply. Clients looking for help in counseling centers are not primarily those who have to endure unbearable sufferings rooted in the past or experienced in the present, but those who don't know what to do with their lives. They have no goal to struggle for because they see no values worth living—much less sacrificing—for. Their lives are empty. They are bored, frustrated, and anxious.

Frankl's picture of the human being includes the human spirit, the noëtic dimension, which is still largely ignored in therapy, just as the psychological dimension was ignored in the early days of Freud.

The inclusion of the human spirit does not mean that we are to deny our animal drives and emotions, or our desire to be successful and materially secure. But it does mean the acknowledgment of a dimension in which we are free to decide whether to give in to our impulses or to resist them. The spirit is the dimension in which a potential murderer, even if provoked, is able to take a stand against these drives. In this *noëtic* dimension, even severe and unavoidable suffering can be overcome by a change of attitudes that can turn the suffering into a human achievement. When the noëtic dimension is included, human beings are free to deny themselves pleasure if they see meaning behind the denial. Here, they are not dominated by the pleasure principle, but can make decisions according to the meaning principle. Frankl's philosophy and therapy are based on the assumption—increasingly supported by empirical evidence—that the human being is motivated to live and to act not so much by having something to live *on*, but something to live *for*, a task to fulfill, an idea to realize, a goal to reach. These are old truths, intuitively accepted by the person in the street but not yet in psychiatric clinics and counseling centers.

Suppose a mother of two small children, struggling to make a living, is invited to a dream villa on the Riviera where she can loll on the beach and eat lobster and caviar; she will reply, regretfully: "How can I go away? Who will take care of my kids?" This decision cannot be explained by saying she simply follows her motherly instincts, or that she never learned a different behavior than to serve her family. Such explanations devalue her basic humanness by placing her action below the human and spiritual level—an example of a malignant reductionism. What asserts itself here is the will to meaning, the voice of conscience. Her decision goes against the pleasure principle: She would rather be on the beach eating lobster than washing diapers at home. But she has a task to fulfill; she is needed by her children. She would not be able to enjoy her luxuries knowing that the children are at home, unattended.

MOTIVATION IN THE AFFLUENT SOCIETY

In the marketplace of the affluent society, everything can be purchased... except meaning. Industry produces thousands of articles to satisfy the pleasure principle, and life becomes empty. Children sit in their own rooms filled with expensive toys and are bored. Their parents work to afford the new freezer, the second car, and all the luxuries that have become meaningless. The young try to break out of that trap; in their desperate search for some remaining values and ideals, they stumble into drug abuse, violence, terrorism, political excesses, destructive protests, or cults. On weekends, the family rushes to amusement centers; they fly to faraway vacation spots; they never come to a standstill, they never come to their senses, they never quiet down to a conversation that goes much beyond a superficial chat. Television programs either simulate a nonexistent harmony or emphasize

1. Logotherapeutic View of Human Nature

violence. People live apart, they live for themselves, they live without a purpose. Clinics are overcrowded with those who are sick, suffering from the meaninglessness of an affluent life that is rich in material possessions but hardly worth living.

However, there are signs that this affluence has peaked. Perhaps our energy crises, economic crises, and political crises are warning signs that, in order to survive, we need to understand ourselves as human beings that are primarily oriented to meaning. Perhaps the drug of affluence, which we have all swallowed, will help us not to hallucinate but to face reality: Human beings are not primarily concerned with satisfying needs and seeking reinforcements but rather with perceiving and pursuing meaningful goals.

Emotions may often misguide us, but our will can move mountains. Conditioned reflexes may lead us astray, but our intellect can rediscover the right way. We have evolved from animals, but we do possess a uniquely human dimension of the spirit that lifts us above the animal level. Our brain functions like a computer, but our conscience helps us resist any brainwashing or preprogramming.

We are full of contradictions, but the ability to live within these paradoxes is a specifically human quality that enables us to contradict even our drives and our learned behavior, and to overcome our limits, failures, and weaknesses. This self-image presupposes a trust in human nature.

The logotherapeutic picture of the human being is permeated by a trust in our full humanness. It does not reduce human actions to egoistic motives that must be unmasked, or to mechanisms that must be manipulated. Logotherapists recognize human beings in their fullness, including their capacity to suffer, to experience guilt, and to face death. This picture of human nature opens new vistas.

The view that we are able to live fully, in the face of unavoidable suffering, inerasable guilt, and the certainty of death (which Frankl called the *tragic triad*) is a reason for hope, belief, and trust in human nature because it perceives human nature at the highest level.

"Being"—
magical word for an incomprehensible existence,
never fathomed,
never fully perceived,
never completely thought through.

"Being alive"—
magical words of a mysterious nature,
never completed,
never halted in its development,
never aware of its goal.

"Being human"—
magical words of spiritual essence,
never satisfied,
never resting,
always in pursuit of meaning.

Elisabeth Lukas

CHAPTER 2

Logotherapy: Health Through Meaning

Logotherapy (literally, "health through meaning") provides a view of human nature that helps us to regain and to retain our health. It sees us not only as creatures that are shaped by genes, drives, and environment, but also as individuals who can shape ourselves within—and often in spite of—our biological, psychological, and environmental influences.

We can do this because our primary motivation is our will to meaning and because we have the freedom to find meaning moment by moment, either by changing a meaningless situation or by changing our attitude when the situation cannot be changed.

How can we find health through meaning? This approach to health is based on three basic aspects of meaning as the logotherapist sees them.

THREE ASPECTS OF MEANING

The first aspect is that *meaning cannot be arbitrarily chosen*. What is meaningful for one person at a specific moment is not necessarily so for another. For a farmer, the meaning of the moment may be feeding livestock. For a volunteer fireman, it may be to rush to a fire. For the farmer to go and watch the fire, or for the fireman to feed his animals would mean that each might have missed the meaning of the moment.

The meaning of the moment thus has an objective component, contained in a situation not created—at least not exclusively—by the individual. It must always be remembered that meaning is to be discovered by each person and cannot be given or prescribed by another.

The second aspect is that *we cannot be driven to meaning* by conscious or unconscious forces, nor can we find meaning through conditioning. Drives and conditioning factors are found in the realm of subjective gains, such as pleasure, avoidance of pain, all types of positive feedback, and such currently popular goals as self-confirmation, self-finding, and self-actualization. Here, a certain behavior brings subjective gains as a reward.

The objective meaning of a situation lies not in serving the meaning-seeker but in serving another person or a cause. Subjective gain is possible as a by-product. The farmer who feeds his or her livestock does it for the sake of the animals; the volunteer firefighter saves lives and property. Their personal rewards are incidental: more productive animals, possibly saving one's own home from the spreading fire. But personal gain is not the decisive factor. Under certain circumstances the farmer may even risk the lives of the animals to save neighbors from fire.

This leads to the third aspect: *Meaningful actions can result in personal gain, but as a by-product.* Often, the gain is greater the less it is intended. One might modify an old biblical wisdom: He who wants to gain his life will lose it. He who is ready to lose it—to give it up to a meaningful task—will gain it.

To return to our examples: The farmer who disregards all physical, psychological, and environmental handicaps to take care of land and livestock will gain by feeling deeply rooted in his farm. The firefighter who prevents disaster finds fulfillment deepened by the appreciation of others.

Obviously, such actions are meaningful only if directed toward a goal worth the effort, and not if they are meaningless "sacrifices," results of masochistic tendencies, or consequences of the inability to say "no." Meaningful actions are subjective responses to the objective meaning of the moment.

2. Logotherapy: Health Through Meaning

THE LOGOTHERAPEUTIC APPROACH TO HEALTH

The logotherapeutic approach is thus based on these three consequences of Frankl's understanding of meaning: Meaning cannot be arbitrarily chosen, it does not result from drives or conditioning, and its pursuit leads to personal gains only as a by-product. Logotherapy offers help to the psychologically unstable and sick as well as to healthy persons in spiritual distress. It helps individuals in their search for meaning to discover what is most meaningful in their particular life situations.

The use of logotherapy motivates clients to open themselves to meaningful actions and experiences, to entrust themselves to the meaning of the moment, and to say "yes" to what the situation demands. Their recovery, "finding themselves," their inner satisfaction will come as unintended by-products—treasures carried by the current of meaning fulfillment, inaccessible when the current loses strength.

The goal of logotherapy is to stimulate the flow of meaning fulfillment in individuals, to guide them to *surrender* to this flow, one that carries all that makes life worth living. These goals underlie the practice of logotherapy.

How logotherapy works in practice fills whole libraries. In this chapter, I shall limit myself to four polarities in human life, the basis of interpretation and application in all schools of psychotherapy including logotherapy: conscious vs unconscious, past vs future, positive vs negative, the want vs the ought.

CONSCIOUS VS UNCONSCIOUS

In general, logotherapy focuses on the individual's conscious understanding. When something unconscious is lifted into the conscious, it is more often from that which is not conscious in the noëtic dimension (the human spirit), and not so much from the unconscious of the psychic dimension (the emotions and intellect). An example will clarify the distinction.

Ms. P suffered from depression. A long psychoanalysis uncovered hidden connections and unconscious threads buried in her past, but her depression deepened. She wanted to try a different therapeutic approach.

Her problem was age-old: Married to a good husband, with a healthy child she loved, she fell in love with another man. In a conflict of conscience she went to a therapist who, in long hours, revealed that she was the victim of a series of projections: She was not really in love with the other man, but unconsciously projected onto him her secret wishes that were not fulfilled by either her father or her husband. It was this that made the other man so attractive and desirable. Were she to live with him, these projections would collapse like a house of cards and she would face bitter disappointment. The therapist advised her to bring up to her consciousness all those wishes and needs that father and husband left unfulfilled, to freely vent her anger, and to force her father and her husband to fulfill her wishes.

In theory, of course, there may be some truth in this interpretation but, in practice, in the noëtic dimension Ms. P suffered something that could be called a *loss of values*. When she explored with the psychoanalyst the "debts" her father and her husband owed her for not fulfilling her needs, she experienced a devaluation of her relationships with them—relationships that had been basically good. And by converting her love for the other man into a fantasy projection, she experienced a devaluation of her genuine feelings for him. What remained was dissatisfaction in every respect, resulting in a long-lasting depression.

With logotherapy, we chose a different approach. I started with her conflict of conscience, between her original "yes" to her husband and the new "yes" to her friend, all seemingly having little to do with her father. She had to make an inner decision, not between conscious and unconscious wishes but a decision that was *meaningful*—meaningful *for all persons involved*.

To help Ms. P with her decision, I asked her to tell me something about these four people: husband, child, friend, and herself. My interest was focused on what made each of these persons unique and irreplaceable, what made them especially lovable.

It turned out that she had a lot to say about her husband and child, but hesitated in talking about herself and her friend. She had changed a lot since her affair, she said, and the other man was difficult to describe. She really didn't know much about him. She loved him but wondered if

2. Logotherapy: Health Through Meaning

he deserved her love. Suddenly she added, "And neither do I deserve the love of my husband and my child any longer."

"What would be needed to make your friend and yourself deserving of love?" I asked.

She replied softly: "If we gave each other up."

I was silent, and she remained silent. Then with a faint smile, she said:

> Yes, it suddenly came to me. For all four to remain deserving of love, my friend and I would have to separate while we still loved each other. I'd keep him in good memory, my husband would appreciate me again, it would save my child much grief, and I could face myself. I really think I have to come to an understanding with my friend about this, or none of us will deserve any love. We'd continuously blame each other.

It was not easy for Ms. P to give up her friend, but the depression dissipated immediately. My explanation is that her decision, in the noëtic dimension, brought about a *gain of value*: Her family gained value by the renewal of her original "yes," and genuine love for her friend was not devaluated as a fantasy projection but gained value through freely giving it up.

In dealing with value conflicts, logotherapists do not transfer their own values to patients. It is true that in every interpersonal communication, each partner unavoidably transmits something of his own value system to the other. But logotherapists are protected from such transference because they help their patients weigh conflicting values in relation to the objective meaning of the moment.

To use a metaphor, one might say that logotherapists free the two balls brought by the patient from all extraneous wrappings until it becomes clear which is lead and which is gold. Therapist and patient face the same set of undeniable facts, just as the meaningfulness of a situation is also undeniable once recognized. The therapist does not declare one value as higher. It is not the therapist's brush that paints the ball gold; it is the inner core of the value itself that is the determining factor, enabling each person to use a given situation in the best possible way.

It is true that our Socratic dialogue did lift something from Ms. P's unconscious into the conscious: her responsibility toward the three whose lives were significantly influenced by her decision.

THE PAST AND THE FUTURE

On the whole, logotherapy focuses on possibilities that lie in the future. However, introspection is not avoided; for example, in experiences that haven't been worked through that require a more meaningful attitude in the present, or when a life nears its end and requires reflection. What logotherapists do *not* look for in the past are causes for present unwanted behavior, because they do not believe human behavior is completely determined by psychosocial or psychophysical causes. In the specifically human dimension, we adopt an attitude to all causes that may condition us, and this is an "unconditional" factor that is not predetermined, but based on free will.

For this reason, the practitioner of logotherapy does not regard parental mistakes as sufficient reason for developmental problems in the psyches of children. Mistakes by parents can be corrected by grown children through self-education, if they so desire. Individuals with neurotic symptoms, however, often do not want to correct anything; rather, they use their symptoms to accuse the "guilty" parents. I remember one patient who said triumphantly: "Yes, I could behave normally… but if I do that, the brutality of my parents will not show any negative consequences, and I don't want that to happen. The world should see what they did to me, so they will suffer."

This patient, with sadistic tendencies, had to be shown the contradiction in her own words. If it was up to her to behave normally or abnormally, as she herself stated, there could be no one else responsible for her normal or abnormal behavior.

Professionals, too, often get trapped in this contradiction, which shows how difficult it is to distinguish between the freedom we have in the noëtic dimension and our fate—the lack of freedom we experience in body and psyche. This was demonstrated at a drug addiction conference. Many speakers argued that lack of maternal love in early childhood, refusal of

2. Logotherapy: Health Through Meaning

breast feeding, exclusion of children from family life, lack of body contact, and so on drive the children later to drugs. An Italian pediatrician pointed out that Italian children receive love from babyhood on and are a close part of the family, yet drug addiction in Italy is especially high. "Our experience in Italy," he concluded, "contradicts all your theories." No one on the panel of experts knew the answer.

Logotherapists, at least, have a suggestion. Without underestimating the importance of the past, the theory of logotherapy puts forth the idea that aspects of the future play an equal, or perhaps even a greater, part. If young people see no meaningful realistic goals, no ideals, no commitments, nothing to achieve in their youthful enthusiasm, then there is nothing to prevent them from escaping into artificial meanings, intoxication, and self-destruction.

I experienced the close connection between this feeling of meaninglessness and self-destruction with a young patient. She told me she walked almost daily along railroad tracks. "If I had the courage," she said, "I'd throw myself in front of a train. Then I would be free from all broodings and doubts of what I am here for."

I struggled with her in the noëtic dimension of her spirit. "Yes," I said, "you would be free *from* something but no longer free *for* something. Throwing yourself in front of a train would free you from feelings of meaninglessness, but you'd no longer be free to make something meaningful of your life. A meaningless death would not enrich your life with meaning. You would have bought your freedom *from* at the price of your freedom *for*."

I asked her to describe her daily path to the tracks. It passed a crossroad; to the right, it led to the railroad; to the left, the forest. I told her:

> Next time you come to the crossroad, stop for a moment and taste the freedom you have. You can choose between left and right, yes or no, between the two directions. You can weigh possibilities and choose the meaningful. To have this specifically human freedom makes life worth living. One disastrous step, and you no longer have this freedom to weigh and choose, not even the freedom to take back your step.

What requires courage is not the step onto the tracks, but the step into the quiet forest, where you can sit down and think about the tasks awaiting you, including those perhaps only you can fulfill. When you come to the crossroad next time, will you stop and think about this?

She did think about it, and eventually decided to resume training as a pediatric nurse, which has been interrupted because of domestic trouble.

The past has power only where no future is visible.

THE POSITIVE AND THE NEGATIVE

Practitioners of logotherapy tend to focus on the positive, even in the presence of negative factors. This helps clients to see and to promote the positive, accentuating achievement over failure. Even in the diagnostic phase, this stance is obvious. Here, the logotherapist's aim is not to make clients recall painful, repressed experiences but rather to remember forgotten highlights, to refurbish them in a manner that outshines present troubles.

The therapeutic phase also emphasizes the positive, and thus helps individuals find a positive attitude and necessary acceptance in the face of incurable physical or psychological illnesses. For curable illness, however, acceptance is neither needed nor desirable because it prevents patients from resisting the illness.

This is also true for phobias, obsessive compulsions, and sexual neuroses, all triggered by the mechanism of *anticipatory anxiety*, trapping patients in a vicious cycle. Such patients anticipate something negative, and consequently something negative happens, at least in their heads, and often in reality, reinforcing the negative anticipation that brings about whatever is feared.

One example is sexual dysfunctions. People afraid of failure in entering a situation of intimacy hardly have a chance. Anxiety causes physical tension, distracts attention from the partner, and leads to observing themselves and their sexual performance, which prevents surrender to the partner. But this self-surrender is exactly what is needed to bring about happiness and pleasure as a by-product. This is also true of surrender to a *logos incarnate*,

2. Logotherapy: Health Through Meaning

as Frankl called the specifically human love that finds physical expression in the union of two human beings.

To help patients escape this trap, methods of *paradoxical intention* and *dereflection* are useful in logotherapy. A brief case history illustrates them:

Mr. and Ms. M, both middle-aged, found their harmonious marriage disturbed by her tetanic spasms, increasingly frequent. Whenever he approached her romantically she had an attack that made intimacy difficult, and made him suspect that she used her illness as an excuse to reject him. Ms. M denied this but he remained skeptical, leading to quarrels. Ms. M's physicians were not sure about the causes of the spasms, and used the word "psychosomatic."

I explained that the term meant that the illness had a somatic (physical) cause but was triggered by something occurring in the psyche. Tetanic spasms are caused by a shortage of calcium or magnesium in the body, often in connection with a hypoparathyroidism, an underfunctioning parathyroid gland. The shortage shifts the acid-base equilibrium of the body toward the alkaline. This equilibrium can also be disturbed by hyperventilation, over-rapid breathing in which much carbon dioxide is exhaled, which shifts the acid-base equilibrium toward the alkaline. Hyperventilation is often the result of psychic agitation occurring when one anticipates something negative.

Thus when he wants to make love, she has a tetanic spasm caused by a lack of calcium or magnesium. This results in fearfully anticipating a spasm the next time in the same situation. Anticipation triggers hyperventilation, and this, in turn, triggers a spasm that would not have happened for lack of calcium or magnesium alone. The vicious cycle of the trap is closed: The husband wants to make love, his approach makes her fear a spasm, anticipatory anxiety triggers hyperventilation, the spasm confirms the anticipatory fear, and her behavior confirms his suspicion that she "manufactures" spasms when he wants to make love, and he doubts her love.

After I explained to the couple the interrelationship between body and psyche, we entered the noëtic dimension of the human spirit where a person, if need be, can say "no" to anxieties and doubts. Using paradoxical intention, I recommended to the husband that he show her gentle affection without intention for intercourse. This behavior would reduce her anticipatory anxiety. At the same time, I suggested to the wife, using the technique of dereflection, not to think about spasms but about qualities she loved in her husband. She might even try to take the initiative for intercourse, when he showed no intention. We thus reversed roles: She was to become the gentle aggressor while he was instructed to refrain from intercourse.

They found my suggestions strange but obviously tried because at the next counseling session he admitted with embarrassment to successful intercourse. "I really wanted to apply the brakes," he said, "but then…."

She added: "It really happened the way you said. I concentrated on my husband and remembered when we first met, and that we still loved each other. I forgot my sickness and everything, and suddenly we were in each other's arms, with no tension of spasms. I am happy to know this is still possible."

Since then, the tetanic attacks have been reduced to a minimum and probably will not require medical or psychotherapeutic help. The marriage is proceeding normally, which proves that the positive is possible even in those situations in which the negative exists.

THE WANT VS THE OUGHT

The "ought" is the ethical directive, how our personal conscience tells us to act in response to the meaning of the moment, to make us aware that what we feel deep within us is most meaningful. If the "want" is the result of our will to meaning, it is in accord with the ought because both are oriented toward meaning, and no bad consequences will follow. But if the want is the result of another will (such as the will to pleasure or the will to power), or the ought is superimposed on us by outside influences (parents, peers, society) and does not lead us to respond to the meaning of the moment as we see it, then there is a gap between the ought and the want that may cause considerable psychological conflict. Therefore, the task of the therapist is to bring the ought and the want together.

2. Logotherapy: Health Through Meaning

For instance, when parents spoil and overprotect their children, the therapist may argue that the most meaningful way to raise children is to do what is best for their physical-psychological-spiritual upbringing. This is the ought. But for most normal parents, it is also the want. On this basis, the therapist may discuss with parents how refraining from spoiling and overprotecting contributes to the well-being of the child.

There are also examples demonstrating that a personal want, directed toward a meaningful goal, is at the same time an ought that must not be prevented by outside forces. The want and the ought of a person can harmonize only if both relate to meaning, even though one demands a decision and the other is a request.

Every want requires a decision in favor of what is wanted (for instance, painting); every ought is a request to refuse what ought not to be (for instance, spoiling a child).

Logotherapy deals with both the want and the ought, and tries to harmonize them toward an objective meaning. In this manner, logotherapy stands in contrast to most other schools of psychotherapy, which focus attention on what is wanted, especially in the intrapsychic area of human drives, and less in the area of trans-subjective meaning.

RATIONALITY AND EMOTION

A meta-analysis was used to compare effectiveness of various types of psychotherapy using around 500 empirical studies. Glass and Kliegle (1983) concluded:

> Most effective proved to be cognitive methods of therapy which were based on rational confrontation with the convictions and thoughts of the patients. Second most effective were methods using hypnosis to bring about changes in the patients' experiences and behavior patterns.
>
> Methods in behavior therapy, aimed, for instance, at self-control or training in certain abilities, were third, followed by the treatment of certain phobias through systematic desensitization. Other forms of therapy proved to be less

effective, such as psychoanalytically oriented therapies, Gestalt- and client-centered therapy. (pp. 29-31) [1]

Because this meta-analysis was open to criticism for its methods, Klaus Grawe of the University of Bern, Switzerland, checked the effectiveness of the various psychotherapies in a more detailed study. In an unpublished report he concluded:

> Preliminary results of a detailed examination of some 1,000 international studies of psychotherapies by the Bern research team found humanistic methods the most effective. These include therapies emphasizing the experience and stimulation of emotions and meaning aspects. Behavior therapy and psychoanalytically oriented treatments followed at a significant distance.

These findings are quoted not to disparage other psychotherapies but to point out the potential effectiveness of logotherapy. According to the meta-analysis, the most effective methods were "based on rational confrontation with the convictions and thoughts of the patients." The Bern research team declared as most effective "humanistic methods... therapies emphasizing the experience and stimulation of emotions and meaning aspects." Effective methods, therefore, appeal to both a) a rationale confronting patients' convictions and b) the evocation of emotions that are oriented toward meaning. This is exactly the combination stimulated by logotherapeutic dialogue: on rational thinking and acting—not rigid, but based on deep-rooted values and ethical convictions; and on active emotions—not focused on self, but transcending self toward persons and causes that are meaningful.

Logotherapy is not just *a* humanistic method, it is possibly *the* humanistic method because its goal is an appeal to what is *specifically human* in every person: It helps patients regain their full human capacities. Professionals

---

[1] Glass, G. V., & Kliegl, R. (1983). An apology for research integration in the study of psychotherapy. *Journal of Consulting & Clinical Psychology, 51*(1), 28-41. [Lukas' manuscript was originally written in German, so the research article was translated into German for this quote, then back to English. This abbreviated excerpt of the findings, while not exact, is accurate. At the time of publication, the original article could be accessed at: http://opus.kobv.de/ubp/volltexte/2009/4023/ –Ed.]

2. Logotherapy: Health Through Meaning

in the helping field may find guidance in the words of Munich surgeon K. H. Bauer: "If science is the rock on which we stand, humanity is the star toward which we reach."

> If you believe
> you always have
> to still your hunger
> before you can think
> of the meaning of life,
> you are mistaken.
>
> Because without knowing
> about the deeper
> meaning of life
> you can bear
> neither hunger
> nor full satiation.
>
> Elisabeth Lukas

CHAPTER 3

What is Special About Logotherapy? A Representation of its Holistic Concept With Narrative Elements

There are currently over 800 psychotherapeutic schools, techniques, and methods which can claim respectability or, in other words, do more than merely defraud suffering people. They can all report certain successes in treatment, even if many of them operate on the level of suggestion or have a mere placebo effect. This does not devalue their successes.

Nevertheless, the calls in recent decades for a holistic approach in the treatment of mental illness have become louder. This is because the various therapies not only have their own intrinsic value, their higher or lower level of quality, but they also all have a starting point of "somewhere" on the person. To be exact, they start at some excerpt—or even directly at some defect—of the human being that they wish to reduce or compensate for.

Autogenic training, for example, one of the most effective relaxation techniques, starts with physical and psychological relaxation of the human being. Catharsis, on the other hand, an old method of emotional release, bases its approach on the person's inhibited state and on the tendency to suppress emotions. Of course, neither of these methods asks whether tension or self-control are perhaps entirely appropriate in each case. In other words, whether a certain method begins at the right time and at the correct psychological state of a patient is not apparent until we arrive at a metalevel, a level that transcends the mere listing of descriptions of illnesses and corresponding treatments and includes the essence of being human—the noëtic—as something that is much more than the sum of symptoms.

For consideration on this metalevel, a truly holistic psychotherapy is necessary, one free of the notion of rundown psychological mechanisms in need of repair, one that moves forward to the mysteriously winding ways that carry the seeds of fulfillment because they orient themselves on human nature. Thus the explosion of theoretical stances in the helping professions has led to a counterreaction in the form of a search for a plain, simple understanding, for a sort of inner clarity that is concerned mainly with that which is essential to life. This could yield the recognition and defusing of impulses that cause illness as a by-product, without making them its primary concern.

Viktor Frankl's logotherapy is the first successful creation of such a truly holistic psychotherapy. How do I know this? Simply because the logotherapeutic viewpoint begins with a whole: the world. The whole cannot be grasped by us humans, not even with the help of all the sciences. Therefore, logotherapy brings human existentiality into play, manifested in the intuitions and sensing of all peoples and generations—concealed in a thousand symbols and rites—with a growing realization that the whole must have some kind of ultimate meaning behind it that goes beyond chaos and chance. In this famous text passage, Frankl noted:

> The question is: "Is existence nothing but a mass of nonsense, or is it a mass of ultimate meaning?" This question cannot be answered by the natural sciences alone. It cannot be answered at all, it is a completely unsolvable problem—rather, it must be decided. All being is ambiguous: both interpretations—both the interpretation "nonsense" and the interpretation "ultimate meaning"—are possible. Both are thinkable: that being is total nonsense, and that it is total ultimate meaning; but these are indeed only two "thinkables," two thought possibilities,

3. What is Special About Logotherapy?

and not thought necessities. With respect to the decision we are called upon to make, there is no logical coercion; in no way are we logically forced, logically obligated to decide for one or the other. Both interpretations are logically of equal status. Logically there is as much which speaks for the one interpretation as for the other. The equal status of the two answers: the answer "absolute nonsense" and the answer "absolute ultimate meaning"—results in the responsibility of the respondent. He is not only faced with a question—No: He is faced with a decision, and, in fact, an existential decision, but not an intellectual decision. What he must perform is not the "intelligere," not a factual realization—but rather a personal commitment.

Reasons and objections are balanced as on a set of scales, but the decision maker throws the weight of his own being onto one side of the scales.

It is not knowledge which makes this decision, but rather faith; but *faith is not thinking minus the reality of that which is thought, but rather thinking, enriched by the existentiality of the thinker* [emphasis added].[1]

This is at the same time the "primal therapeutic act" that logotherapy carries out and presents for the purpose of imitation in its treatment concept. It is throwing one's own "yes" onto one side of the scales that swing back and forth in the incomprehensible, onto the side that knows about the meaning of the whole and believes in it.

Only the "yes," the personal commitment, as Frankl emphasized, the weight of the being of the person, who pronounces his or her "yes," allows the chosen side of the scales to weigh more than the other side, which knows nothing of the meaning of the whole and does not believe in it. Both are intellectually thinkable, but the chosen side is enhanced by the existentiality of the thinker—and thus sinks lower, outweighing the other. It is this side, along with its core content, which will henceforth count. The great nonsense of the whole as a troubling last resort which would ban

---

1 Frankl, V. E. (1993). *Der Mensch vor der Frage nach dem Sinn, 9th ed.* Munich: Piper, p. 274.

all striving and effort into the absurd will no longer hinder the unfolding of this human life.

The "primal therapeutic act" therefore consists of coupling being and meaning. And there is no treatment and no support of a suffering person that can do without it. For where being is not coupled with meaning, human health, happiness, bravery, etc. have no meaning. In fact, therapy would be pointless. All values would then be merely human evaluations and could be cancelled again by human evaluations. Even the value "patient" would be only a fiction pertaining to a meaningless heap of matter. And the value "recovery of the patient" would also amount to an equally arbitrary subjective judgement. It would then be, in objective terms, a matter of indifference, whether the world exists or not, whether people, animals, plants, cultural achievements, continue to exist—their being would not be any better than their nonbeing, their preservation not better than their destruction. Without the "yes" to the opponent of blind evolutionary chance—namely to a *logos-ness* of the world, which, in principle, grants "being" the title *ought-to-be*—therapeutic activity has no foundation.

Thus we can say that logotherapy begins with the whole, even with the meaning of the whole, with the scientifically unprovable meaning: "In the beginning was the logos"[1] to quote one of Frankl's German books. This and no less than this is the metalevel from which logotherapy has been developed. It is a system that makes use of scientific method, but nevertheless must bear the burden of the unprovability of its—existential—starting point. I wish to demonstrate with three aspects how fruitfully this thought system, with its widely varied consequences for psychological practice, is carried by its holistic approach.

1) FROM THE MEANING OF THE WHOLE FOLLOWS THE MEANING OF ALL OF ITS PARTS

If being as a whole has meaning, then everything that is must be imbued with meaning, right down to the "mini-unit" of a quiet hour. Then and only then does every human life have meaning: every tree, every sunrise,

---

1 Frankl, V. E. (1994). *Im Anfang war der Sinn*, 3rd ed. Munich: Piper.

3. What is Special About Logotherapy?

every melody, every smile, and every joy. Then, however, every inevitable sorrow also has its meaning, along with every effort, every step toward maturity, every act of growth, every wrongdoing, and every resurrection. Under the roof of the great, all-encompassing ultimate meaning, even the small, tender, rejected thing blooms in far-from-negligible significance.

This provides an argumentative opening for the widespread lack of self-worth problematic of the many patients in psychotherapy who do not know their own worth, do not value it, or do not affirm it—those who do not explore their freedom, grow their abilities, who are not aware of their deepest feelings, and consider themselves completely superfluous… those who simply make nothing of their lives.

Why not? Because they do understand themselves as partial being within being as a whole, but not as partial meaning within the greater meaning of the whole. The message that "You are important, you are needed, all your experiences are important, even the painful ones, because they qualify you for a special task, which only you can fulfill…" can be communicated only in the context of a world perceived to have a meaningful structure, a world in which every person is specifically *intended*: intended as a new hope which arrives in the world like the dawn of a new day of creation in the history of the living.

On this theme, a fable by the Arab mystic Sa'di[1] titled "The tiger and the disabled fox":

> On the way through the forest a man saw a fox who had lost its legs. He wondered how the animal could survive. Then he saw a tiger with its kill. The tiger had eaten enough and left the rest for the fox.
>
> On the next day God nourished the fox again with the help of the same tiger. The man was astonished at God's great goodness and said to himself: "I, too, will rest in a corner and place my full trust in God, and he will provide for all my needs."

---

1 Cited in de Mello, A. (1998). *Warum der Vogel singt*. Freiburg: Herder, p. 64; for the original English edition, see de Mello, A. (1984). *The song of the bird*. New York: Image Doubleday, pp. 79-80.

He spent many days in this way, but nothing happened, and the poor fellow was near death when he heard a voice: "You there, on the wrong path, open your eyes to the truth! Follow the example of the tiger, and stop imitating the disabled fox."

The man crept out of his corner. On the road he met a small girl, shivering with cold in a thin dress, with no hope of getting anything warm to eat. He became angry and said to God: "How can you permit this? Why do you not act?"

For a while God said nothing. But in the night he suddenly answered: "I did do something about it. I created you."

Here we have the world with a meaningful structure, in which everything has its meaningful place: the fox and the tiger, the man and the girl, the loss of legs and the successful hunt, questions and answers, error and insight. The fable focuses on the man, however, because he has not yet found his meaningful place. Like so many patients in psychotherapy, his eyes have not been opened to the truth.

What truth eludes him? The truth of the tiger, who also provides for the fox. The truth of the tiger, who is not there for himself alone, but rather fulfills meaning in interaction with the world. Without doubt, the fox has its tasks, but here what matters is clearly the example of the tiger, which "the man on the wrong path" does not follow. The story is about giving, sharing, involving oneself, about that which is demanded of, and assigned to, every one of us on, our own responsibility.

"Follow the example of the tiger…"—often, logotherapy is nothing but the psychotherapeutic translation of this appeal: "Do not ask what has been done to you. Do not ask what someone will do for you. Ask instead what you can do. Do not wait for someone to take care of you, but, instead take care of something yourself. Do not complain about conditions where you are and do not rail at God and your fate. Something has been done about it: You were created. You have been placed in the path of a shivering girl, just as the tiger was placed near the fox. So come out of the corner in which your life has been taking its empty course, where you have been slowly approaching psychological decline, and take on what is yours. Then

3. What is Special About Logotherapy?

you will become healthy. And should you get into difficulty at some time, fear not! Someone has also been created who has been placed on your path, if you really need it...."

This approximates the logotherapeutic approach called the *evocation of the will to meaning*. The method of dereflection applies it in countless variations. It constantly draws the attention of the patient to the shivering, hungry girl, in whatever form she may appear: as a person in need of comfort, a matter to be taken care of, a work to be completed.

She is there, she is in his road, in need of his advance pledge in love. The devoted service to her, to which the patient will rise, will cure his soul. Not the therapy from outside—but rather his own love—will heal him. What the therapy can achieve is merely a strengthening of his ability to go beyond himself, just the opening of his spiritual eyes.

One thing is clear in all of this: If the whole had no meaning, no meaning could be found in the details. The fox would have been out of luck, and the tiger would have been stupid not to eat his own prey. The man in the corner would have received no instructions, and the girl's shivering with cold would not have been his business. Therapeutically, one could advise the man that he follow his drive to seek nourishment, just as the tiger kills its prey, but beyond the fulfillment of basic needs, no inherent "creative value" could be activated that would raise him to the level of a "co-creator." We would have the side of the scales in which, instead of the lost legs of the fox, a lost world would lie, lost in the indifference of chaos.

2) FROM THE MEANING OF THE WHOLE FOLLOWS THE ASSUMPTION OF PERMANENCE

If being as a whole has meaning, its end result cannot be nothingness. For with passing, dissolving, eradication of being, the existence of meaning would also pass, and transient meaning would be as good as no meaning. Consequently, being cannot be understood exclusively in the perspective of a return to nonbeing. There must be a reality beyond perishable, destructible matter, which contains something lasting and indestructible; in other words, something eternal in the sense of meaning.

This gives rise to thoughts on the well-known life-and-death fears of patients in psychotherapy, who constantly fear for their scrap of self, because they experience it as easily damaged and totally subject to attack. These are individuals who, blinded by their fears and trapped in their timidity, allow life's great opportunities to pass them by, and later, as their life nears its end, apathetically mourn what they have missed. They have never really been themselves.

To make plain to them that their spiritual core is indestructible, that that which is human persists, even when illness and death cast their shadows, means encouraging them to dare to undertake life. It must also be made plain to them that whatever decision they make, whatever action they perform or fail to perform, flows into the reservoir of the past, in which everything is permanently preserved—but also unchangeably determined—because it can never again be extracted from the truth. This means reminding them to live their lives responsibly. This anthropological fulcrum is nevertheless possible only on the basis of a world that transcends materiality, in which what has been achieved *has been achieved once and for all*, and what has been achieved meaningfully *has eternal meaning*.

On this theme, a story by Pierre Lefevre[1] titled "Knowing the right way":

A sultan dreamed that he was losing all of his teeth. As soon as he woke, he asked an interpreter of dreams what it meant. "Ah, what a misfortune, sire!," he called out. "Every lost tooth means the loss of a family member."

"What, you saucy fellow," the sultan screamed. "What do you dare say to me? Away with you!" And he ordered, "Fifty lashes for this impudence!"

Another interpreter of dreams was called and led before the sultan. When he heard the dream, he called: "What good fortune! Our lord will outlive his whole clan!"

The sultan's face brightened and he said, "Thank you, my friend. Go to my treasurer and have him give you fifty pieces of gold."

---

1 Lefevre, P. (1994). *Aus dem Leben lernen*, *(2nd ed.)* Leutesdorf: Johannes Verlag, p. 32.

3. What is Special About Logotherapy?

> On the way, the treasurer said to the interpreter of dreams, "You didn't interpret the dream any differently than the first interpreter!"
>
> With a sly smile the man replied, "Remember, one can say many things; it depends only on how you say it...."

The story contains two pieces of wisdom. For one, it tells of the dialectic of staying and passing. If I want to remain as the survivor in my family, I must accept the loss of my loved ones. If I do not want to lose my loved ones, I must depart this life before them. Staying is not possible without loss; staying has its price. And that can be generalized: It is only the transitoriness of life that makes life meaningful; only through death does the meaning of a human life remain in existence.

Were life of unlimited duration, every meaningful action could be postponed indefinitely and every meaningless action could be corrected infinitely often,[1] which would mean that human life would move along in an endless grey zone between meaning and countermeaning, never completed in definitive relevance to meaning. If we reasonably want the meaning of a life which is lived to remain in the truth, then we must accept that it will become part of truth with beginning and end, birth and death.

The second piece of wisdom is that the story tells us something about the point of view of facts. "One can say many things, it just depends how...." One can also look at many things, and it depends on how. Logotherapy is often nothing but the correction of a "how" in a patient's viewpoint. The future will bring fifty lashes or fifty gold pieces. It will reward or punish the person for the views and attitudes chosen—attitudes to the same situations!

For the attitude: "Why should I take care of my children? No one took care of me!" it will strike such an individual 20 years later when the great distance to his or her children causes great pain. For the attitude "I suffered as a child, so I want to spare my children that lot!" it will place something precious into that person's hands 20 years later, when the children give warm greetings.

---

1 Frankl, V. E. (1982). *Ärztliche Seelsorge, (10th ed.)* [*The doctor and the soul*]. Vienna: Deuticke, p. 82 ff].

The patient's past, his or her own childhood, cannot be changed, not by any therapeutic intervention, just as the dream of the sultan does not change from one interpreter to the next. But each individual will shape the present differently through a positively changed point of view; it will be shaped more responsibly, more meaningfully, with more orientation to the future.

This is the aim of the therapeutic impulse known in logotherapy as *mobilizing the defiant power of the human spirit*. The method of *attitude modulation* is based on this, in that it helps individuals to perceive aspects of themselves in a new light. This is a method that would lose a great deal of its efficacy if it were linked only to an expectation of a future reward. It derives its efficacy much more from the recognition given to the patient that the actual golden treasure to be gained in life is the lasting value in the truth, the truth about oneself.

3) FROM THE MEANING OF THE WHOLE FOLLOWS INVOLVEMENT IN RELATIONSHIPS

If being as a whole has meaning, then not only all that is must have meaning, but also that which vibrates between that which is, joining things which are. For if the connections between partial meanings were meaningless, they could never join together to form a meaningful whole. Expressed more simply: If a thing is meaningful, then interest in it must also be meaningful, whereby the Latin phrase *inter esse* translates as "that which is between (several being things in a relationship)." From logos follows dia-logue.

The relevance of this dialogue aspect of a meaning-structured world for the relationship crises and self-centeredness of patients treated in psychotherapy is obvious. Many patients live in permanent conflict, even if their conflict partners change, or they refuse contact of every kind, although they are close to suffocating on their loneliness. With family members, coworkers, and acquaintances they do not have an orientation to others but instead curl into a ball in a narcissistic search for illusory self-actualization. If one attempts to open them to their fellow human beings, one often meets

3. What is Special About Logotherapy?

an obstacle. These individuals often have pathological, traumatic contact experiences, and have become distrustful and oversensitive. They do not want to risk rejection. They want guarantees of affection that do not exist. Therefore, they need to understand that every satisfactory relationship requires advance investments, and that these investments must be purely for the sake of the value of the person encountered and not as a payment for something in return. In understanding this, however, they can succeed only through a Weltanschauung that ascribes meaning to mutual attachment itself, whether material or personal.

On this subject, a report from the developmental work of Ernst Lange (abridged), titled "The mud sparrow":[1]

> We were working in a very poor settlement. The people lived in shanties that were so run-down the rain poured in and the wind whistled through them. We had therefore decided to work with them to repair their huts somewhat, so that they would not be cold or even freeze to death in the winter.
>
> One day, Peggy, an American, came to us to help us with the work. Peggy was a beautiful young woman who always looked as if she had just taken a bath and changed her clothes. When I showed Peggy the settlement, she looked horrified. "Oh," she moaned, "how filthy!"
>
> When we entered one of the huts in which we wanted to work, she was close to turning around at the threshold. The widow who lived with her little boy had been sick for weeks and could no longer care for herself properly. There was a terrible stench. Dirty dishes were piled in the sink. The rubbish bin was overflowing. The floor was covered with refuse. Hundreds of flies swarmed about. And the most pitiful object was the little boy in the bed next to his mother. He was perhaps four years old. His thin little body was clad in rags. His black hair was sticky and matted. Saliva was running out of his mouth.

---

1 Lange, E., in Kuhn, J. (ed.). (1991). *Der Engel leuchtende Spuren, (2nd ed.)* Stuttgart: Quell, p. 85.

He woke as we approached. His gaze was immediately fixed on Peggy. "Aunty," he said, as if enchanted. He had probably never seen anything as beautiful as Peggy. He slid off the bed and ran toward her with outstretched arms. I saw her turn as white as death.

"No," she said, "No!" and retreated. But the boy continued, obviously wanting to hug her. "Go away!" screamed Peggy. And when the boy came nearer, she gave him a hard push, so that he fell backwards and began to cry bitterly.

Peggy ran away. I did not catch up with her until I got back to the camp. She was packing her cases. "But Peggy," I said, "you're not serious." "Yes, I am," she said. "I'm leaving. I can't stand it. It's too disgusting." She then took her cases and left as if she couldn't stand being with us a minute longer.

I followed her. I took her cases and made to accompany her to the station. The way led past the house in which we had just been. We saw the boy from a great distance. He was sitting outside watching the cars drive past. "Come on," said Peggy, horrified. "Come, fast." And she went on as fast as she could. But the little boy had already seen us. "Aunty," he shouted, and again spread his little arms. "Aunty!"

Then Peggy was rooted to the spot. "My God," she said. "And I hurt him. I hurt him!" Then everything happened quickly. They began at the same time to run toward one another. In the middle of the street, Peggy stooped down and caught the boy in her arms. A car skidded to a stop a few feet from them. It was a strange picture. The beautiful, elegantly dressed young woman holding the dirty boy in her arms, kissing him, and the driver, too bemused to get angry. I pushed Peggy onto the sidewalk. "What should I do now with your cases?" I asked.

"Perhaps you could take them home again" she answered. "I'll clean up this mud sparrow in the meantime."

The report tells us of something monstrous. Not of the merciful sympathy of a strong tiger for an disabled fox, as in the first story. No, it tells us of the heroism of an disabled fox! For that is what the mud sparrow

3. What is Special About Logotherapy?

is in the report: handicapped, disabled. The filth, a symbol for the misery into which he was born, prevents him from living a healthy, normal life. But it does not prevent him from fulfilling meaning in this world. The boy creates a meaningful relationship between things that are. And he does this spontaneously! This is his heroism, which fully outshines the behavior of the other participants.

But how does he do it? It is important for clients and students of logotherapy to learn this, for the "filth" of their origins and of the circumstances under which they grew up also clings to many of them. Now, the boy does not pay the world back in kind. He does not repay the world at all. He does not bear a grudge, he seeks no revenge, throws no stones, and does not run away. What he radiates is unsoiled. He spreads his arms and runs toward the young woman who rejected him. It is that simple and that incredible. He gives the miracle a second chance—and the miracle happens. A human encounter takes place, not in the shanty, where it belonged, but rather on the street, where it had nearly rushed past. The four-year-old boy rescued it for himself and the woman. The car—the imminent danger—stops; the encounter of the two is blessed.

This is an example of the logotherapeutic impulse that we in logotherapy paraphrase as the *response character of human existence*. We cannot choose the questions life poses to us, but we can choose our responses to them. By means of the method of paradoxical intention, patients learn to put a distance between themselves and their negative experiences and, paradoxically, to approach that which they fear. Thus they give themselves and that with which they have negative associations or expectations the chance of a joint new start. They learn to encounter the world with their best answers, and the world thanks them by taking them into its arms and integrating them into human society.

This kind of autonomy in responding could not be called up if that which oscillates between meaningful things did not have meaning. Were the mud sparrow meaningful only for himself, he would do better to hide from the woman. Were she meaningful only for herself, she would do better to leave the dirty village. Because that which oscillates between the two has meaning, however, the paradoxical sacrifice of the two in going toward one another is the solution of the tragedy, the healing of the soul… a recipe for humanity!

We see that the three aspects which have their foundations in the holistic approach of logotherapy are reflected in its therapeutic methodology and argumentation. Because the whole has meaning, every part has meaning—to be human means *to be intended*. Because the whole has meaning, there is lasting meaning—to be human means *to be effective*. Because the whole has meaning, its relationships have meaning—to be human means *to be involved*. The diagnostic process is nothing but registering where human life deviates from this, its design, and shuts itself off from its existential roots; where it does not take on its tasks, does not fill its place, sees itself as totally vulnerable and destructible, feels superfluous and worthless; where it defines itself as helplessly delivered unto nothingness, powerless, incapable of acting, empty, desperate; where it ends contact, creeps away, runs away, or repays in kind. *And psychotherapy is then nothing but the return of human beings to their natural existence, to the specifically human design, to the image of the logos.*

Of course, psychotherapy must deal with the concrete problems of the individual that, superficially regarded, are much simpler and more unphilosophical. One patient cannot stop smoking, although there is already considerable lung damage; another explodes every time the partner is critical. A third overestimates tenuous business skills again and again and is chronically in debt; a fourth is always afraid to resist manipulation and is always exploited. In order to help these people, it is necessary to have imagination despite all training. The patients' resources must be brought to the fore and their wishes clarified in order to observe their self-perception and assess the steps they are capable of taking toward a better condition.

But the moment comes when the matter gets more philosophical: It transports itself, so to speak, into a larger context. Why work on oneself? Why resist temptation? Why get out of one's rut? Why—and the discussion on meaning has begun. What meaning is there in giving up smoking and living a little longer? What is the meaning of seeking reconciliation with

3. What is Special About Logotherapy?

one's significant other and accepting certain criticisms? What is the meaning in engaging in reasonable business activities and not harming clients? What meaning is there in nurturing one's strength to resist exploitation?

A psychotherapy that is silent on these questions has reached its limits. A psychotherapy that reacts with promises of more pleasure later is laughable. A psychotherapy that replies by throwing onto the scales its conviction of the meaning of the whole, from which every partial meaning is derived, along with the unconditional value and dignity of the human being—including the meaning of all decisions he or she has ever made, in particular any "advance pledges of love," which (with all other decisions) are decisions for eternity—such a psychotherapy is able to stimulate rethinking and renewal.

Such a therapy is logotherapy.

People may be forsaken, lonely,
the loneliness depresses them,
and yet there is
a brilliant
blue
sky.

People may be desperate, sad,
sadness envelops them,
and yet there is
the rich,
warm
earth.

People may be lost, guilty,
guilt is overpowering,
and yet there is
Grace
every-
where.

Elisabeth Lukas

CHAPTER 4

Survival—to What End? Answers to Questions of Fate

Three-and-a-half billion years ago, two different types of life emerged on earth—an event that impacts us today. Around that time, cells came into being that contained chlorophyll, as well as others without it. Regardless of whether or not this happened by coincidence, the fact remains that the possession of chlorophyll determined the ability of the cell to build up its life-giving energy from inorganic material with the help of sunlight, or to be dependent for its sustenance on existing organic substances. Cells with chlorophyll had an advantage because to survive they needed only inorganic material and sunlight, which was in ample supply.

From these cells evolved the chloroplasts that, even today, perform the task of bringing about photosynthesis in the living plant cell, and thus enable plants to survive without capturing and killing other living things. This represents the peaceful life principle existing on earth: the vegetable kingdom.

In contrast, cells lacking chlorophyll needed to kill in order to survive. Unable to convert energy from sunlight for their metabolism, they could survive only at the expense of other life, on which they had to feed in order to receive energy. All animals and humans that have evolved from this cell material inescapably had to follow this aggressive principle of life: They must ingest organic material in order not to starve. To that end, they must hunt, cultivate, and kill organic material—other living things.

Were we to judge rationally these two different life principles, we would doubtlessly come to the conclusion that the aggressive life principle is both biologically disadvantageous and ethically inferior. It depends on the presence of living things which it must incessantly threaten and destroy. And yet, nature in its unfathomable wisdom has come to a different conclusion. It obviously has favored the aggressive over the peaceful life principle, having provided it with senses, the rudiments of consciousness, and finally, with a new and exclusively human dimension: the mind, the spirit, the *noëtic*.

The necessity to destroy is still in us: Even the strictest vegetarian cannot help but eat organic matter in order to survive. But the dimension of the human spirit has opened a new perspective. Our exclusively human, noëtic, dimension can steer aggression, moderate it, guide it into tolerable channels—even take a stand against it. The human spirit can temper the destructive heritage of our cellular foundations through the constructive force of its creativity.

Perhaps it is, after all, not so strange that the aggressive—and not the peaceful—life principle was given the chance to control aggressiveness. Perhaps we can perceive here a glimpse of that mysterious goal toward which evolution unfailingly moves: Everything negative seems somehow and somewhere reversible.

It may seem unusual to regard the dimension of the human spirit as a countermeasure to our biologically inherited principle of destruction. We are inclined to associate the noëtic dimension with the idealized concepts of mind, enlightenment, and imagination. Yet there is ample evidence that the exclusively human dimension of our mind and spirit is not always in accord with our other two dimensions, the *soma* (physical body) and the *psyche* (emotions and intellect); it may even oppose them, acting as a countermeasure. Our mind calls out a "no" when we are inclined toward a "yes," and it may say "yes" when we want a "no." It puts on the brakes when we blindly rush forward, it encourages us when we hesitate, warns us when we err, and makes us strong when we are in danger of becoming weak.

4. Survival—To What End?

Yet, we are still part of the aggressive life principle that genetically forces us to be brutal and self-centered. For a long time, it was thought that animals, at least toward their own kind, are far more tolerant than humans in that they never hurt each other unnecessarily. Recent research has made us more cautious. Not only are the customary fights about sex partners, territory, and food cruel in the animal world, active cannibalism has been observed in 1,300 animal species. For instance, adult crows chop up three-fourths of all crow eggs and newly born crows. There are salamanders that give birth to babies that devour their siblings while still in the womb. A perfect example of the primeval principle of destruction can be found in fish of the genus *Stizostedion* that swallow each other by the tail. Chains of four such fish have been observed that devoured and were devoured at the same time. There is no reason for us humans to ridicule such behavior because in our ways we have created much longer chains of similar madness in our societies. The fight for loot and territory has been imprinted in every single cell of our body since the beginning of time.

On the other hand, nature has given us the exclusive gift of the human spirit, the noëtic dimension, that, in comparison to geological time spans, has existed only for a few moments in the timeline of history. The noëtic dimension has its own laws, which we are just beginning to understand, particularly through research in logotherapy. Spirit does not follow any brutal, egotistic motivations. It requires neither inorganic nor organic material, neither sun nor soil as a source of energy, but material of quite another kind: *Spirit needs meaning*. And because the possibilities of meaning are immeasurable, spirit is limitless. In the form we know it, spirit is still tied to its biological foundations, but essentially it is free. The 3.5 billion-year-old aggressive life principle has merged with a timeless meaning principle.

If we apply this realization to the general practice of psychotherapy, we find traces of both at every step. Every psychological illness is tinged with the touch of destructiveness rooted in our nature; the weak and nonviable has to be eliminated unmercifully in the struggle for survival. Observing the behavior patterns of those who have illness or symptoms of emotional instability, one cannot fail to notice that often they do exactly what is most harmful to themselves. As if driven by an incomprehensible force, they make themselves unhappy. It is painful for the counselor, physician, or therapist to see how much unnecessary suffering patients inflict on themselves; they could lead a normal, fairly unburdened life if they only were a little more calm and content. But these same professional helpers may also witness the converse: People who have been treated cruelly by fate, burdened by undeserved suffering, who grow in the spirit beyond their fate and accomplish deeds of strength far transcending themselves. They see a meaning in their lives and, to fulfill that meaning, acquire added energy to move beyond the circumstances in which they find themselves.

It has been stated that logotherapy is the first school of psychology that includes the phenomena of the spirit in its concept of the human being. I believe this is an understatement. Logotherapy not only includes the phenomena of the spirit; it can also take credit for having discovered the human spirit as a counteragent to the destructive principle within us.

Just as nature has pushed forward from the aggressive life principle to the spiritual meaning principle, so can individual patients suffering from fears, alienation, feelings of inferiority, or symptoms of depression push forward to a triumph of the spirit over their shortcomings. That which we call "evil" does exist in this world and in the hearts of all of us, but since the human being has begun to think, that which we call "good" has become conceivable. Good establishes itself in the struggle to find meaning, which is a simultaneous struggle to find ourselves.

I once had a patient who suffered from a dreadful but unfounded fear of cancer. Several times a day she carefully examined her body for any sign of cancer and this continuous search for deadly symptoms prevented her from living her life. The cancer phobia dominated her completely. The patient was very religious, but her illness made her forget how to pray which, in turn, caused her severe conflicts of conscience because she feared God would punish her with cancer for her silence.

After she had told me that she felt especially bad in the morning and could hardly get up because of her fear, I suggested something that surprised

4. Survival—To What End?

her. I told her to say a short prayer upon waking up: "Dear God, I thank you that I am healthy." While she was full of a subjective fear of cancer, she was to give thanks that, objectively, she was free of cancer. The patient reported later that she could now get up without difficulties and begin her day full of energy. Here the human spirit had acted as a counteragent: The irrational feeling to be sick was countered by the grateful acknowledgment of being healthy. The fear, seen as fate, had been tempered by a trust in an ultimate meaning. This was, of course, only a small part of the recovery process, but it does indicate the usefulness of a logotherapeutic approach.

Next, the patient learned to ridicule her fears. Facing a mirror and looking at her body, she repeated some formulations we had rehearsed: "What? Only one measly cancer is all I have? That's not nearly enough. With my fondness of cancer I'd need at least 10 of them to satisfy me. One alone is a bore!" This nonsense made her laugh, and thus the spell was broken. The more often she was able to trick her phobia in this manner, the less power it had over her, and the less often it tortured her.

Eventually, her symptoms subsided and the time came when I had to guide her back to a normal, healthy life. To achieve this, it was necessary that the mirror in which the woman had anxiously observed herself and her body would symbolically become more and more transparent until it turned into window glass which allowed her to see the world outside. Only when we stop observing ourselves incessantly—and look beyond ourselves at the other things that are meaningful to us—are we cured. If we keep on brooding about ourselves and our small or big problems, we are in as much danger as before; a relapse depends on how much importance we attach to it and to ourselves.

Before the therapy was concluded, our talks no longer dealt with sickness, cancer, and fears. We talked friendships, hikes, taking artistic photographs, about gifts and knitting patterns, learning languages, and airplane trips. The face of the woman relaxed, her motions loosened, her eyes began to smile again. She found new goals to pursue and gained new interests. In addition, we used physical exercises to help her relate positively to her body.

Toward the end of the therapy, she confided in me a minor incident: Recently, she had been struck by the thought that she might develop a sudden stoppage of the bowels after eating certain foods. She told herself: "Now wait a minute, my compulsive obsession now pounces on the bowel area because the horror stories about my cancer don't shock me any more. But I'll put an end to this right away, too!" She made a point to eat all those foods she considered dangerous—and the fear about the stoppage never appeared again. One can imagine how the patient and I enjoyed her victory because no symptom can win against this defiant power of the human spirit; neither can a substitute symptom. This defiant power is an absolute guarantee for stabilization.

This case demonstrates the twofold insight of logotherapy. First, we have resources in our noëtic dimension and, second, these resources can serve as countermeasures to the forces of our soma and psyche. How soma, psyche, and spirit can form a unity while, at the same time, the spirit can, if necessary, distance itself from this unity and rise above it, is a metaphysical mystery. It is an observable fact that in almost every sickness the objective diagnosis and the subjective feeling of the patient affect each other: If the body is sick, the psychological mood is low; if the psyche is sick, the body may develop one or more symptoms. The resources of the spirit, however, need not succumb to illness; they can be activated to resist it. Among the forces of resistance are our capacity for self-distancing and our capacity for self-transcendence, both discovered by logotherapy. We can use them to defy our moods, emotions, confusions, and weaknesses.

When the patient with her cancer phobia managed to ridicule her fear by wishing 10 cancers on herself instead of one, she punctured her neurotic sickness with the resources of her spirit. When, in spite of her condition, she studied English and made travel plans, ignoring her obsession, her spirit took a stand against her illness.

The techniques of paradoxical intention and dereflection that were applied here would never work and result in such amazing successes if they did not contain the fundamental possibility that they, as part of the noëtic dimension, could act as countermeasures.

4. Survival—To What End?

I mentioned the twofold insight of logotherapy, but we must also add a third one, which is perhaps most important. All those resources of mind and spirit that can oppose the biological principle of destruction and individual sickness are not unconditionally available. They, too, require a source of energy: a perception of meaning. It is often stated: "Where there is a will, there is a way." But it's not that simple, as every physician, psychologist, and psychiatrist knows. The will is not enough. The proverb can be formulated in a different way which comes closer to the truth: "We can if we know why we must." Only if there is a *why*, a *what for* behind the will, a will to meaning toward a goal that is so important to us that we make every effort to reach it—only then can the source of energy burst forth from the dimension of the spirit and help us to overcome the feeling and the belief that we cannot.

There are numerous examples that show what human beings are capable of achieving, even when they are sick, old, or disabled, if they have a goal that lends meaning to their efforts. These examples range from mothers who cannot afford to get sick because their small children need them, to criminals who change their old behavior patterns for the sake of someone they love; they include the blind and deaf who, in defiance of their biological handicaps, go beyond what seems possible to achieve, and the dying who extend their biological time span in order to live long enough for some special date or event.

The prevalent research in traditional medicine is focused on determining the role of the psychic dimension (emotions and intellect) in physical illness—without attempting to discover what part the noëtic dimension plays in human health! It is to the credit of logotherapy that we are beginning to see the tremendous and mostly unused possibilities of keeping people healthy by helping them either to find their path to meaning or to ensure that this path at least is not blocked, as happens all too often in highly industrialized countries. Whole libraries of books have been written about the negative influence of disturbed emotions on the organism, but where are the books about the positive influence of the resources of the spirit and the will to meaning upon psyche and body? We know enough about the psychological triggers of illness; the time has come to focus the attention of science on the prevention of sicknesses through the resources of the spirit.

Here is a case in which both play a part. A physician who had worked her entire adult life in a hospital came to see me because of long-standing depressions. Two years earlier, she had serious kidney and stomach surgery. After the operation, she had been given an early retirement. Since then she had taken antidepressants, but her condition worsened. Her will to live flickered and threatened to go out.

I had only one therapeutic session with her, resulting in what Frankl called a "Copernican turnabout" of her mood. What surprised me was the positive effect it had on her physical as well as psychological condition. Not only was her depression lifted, but her health also showed an upswing. The verbatim transcript demonstrates clearly that the mere elucidation of a possible meaning sets in motion the forces of the spirit which had lain fallow: forces that serve as countermeasures to resignation and despair, and thus immunize against many tendencies to illness.

Here is part of our dialogue:

She: I was deeply hurt that my services were terminated because of my sickness.

I: You liked to work in the hospital?

She: Not really, but I'd have never quit on my own.

I: Why not, if you didn't care for it?

She: Well, you know, I always try to do my best. I don't give up easily, regardless of what I do....

I: Wouldn't there be something you'd rather have done than work in a hospital?

She: Yes, I think so. It often bothered me that I didn't have enough time for the patients, everything had to be done in a hurry—from bed to bed—examining patients, giving injections, changing the dressings, checking the temperatures, and then to the next bed, like on a conveyer belt.

4. Survival—To What End?

I: You say you never would have quit your job. What could have made you break away from the hospital to give you the chance to take on a more desirable task?

She: [Thoughtfully] You mean, only through my sickness and my early retirement could I be freed from a job I didn't care for? So I might do something else? I never thought of this before… but come to think of it, it's true.

I: Tell me, when you were very ill, when you were in the intensive care unit facing death, then—as you well know as a physician—much depended on your attitude. Did you want to survive?

She: Yes. Maybe not consciously, but I wanted to survive.

I: If you wanted to go on living, then you must have wanted to live for something. Please try to remember what it was you wanted to survive for? What did you think about in those hours of crisis?

She: I suppose I thought about what a pity it would be if I died now when, in a way, I had not done my best yet—that, so to speak, still lay hidden in me.

I: And now? Your wish came true. You survived. You are liberated from hospital service. You have now what you never had in the hospital: time. Here is your gift: to be alive, to have time. And there is your deep inner need to develop the best in you before it is too late.

She: Strange, listening to you, it almost seems to me as if I have been given a tremendous chance, as if everything had to go that way so this chance could present itself… and I had almost given up my wish to live!

I: All that fight against your sickness, your will to survive—would all this have been worthwhile for an extra time to live if this life would be filled with nothing but emptiness and listlessness?

She: Certainly not. How could I have been so blind! Certainly my life was returned to me to do something with it that makes sense…. And I know what I'd like to do with it. I'd like to comfort lonely people in pain, to do what busy doctors usually have no time for: to sit at the bed of patients and to talk to them, to share their worries and to give them the feeling they are not alone, that someone is with them.

I: You think there are places where you can do this?

She: I think so. I don't need to depend on a salary. In fact, I am not allowed to earn too much in addition to my early pension. I'll ask around in clinics and rehab facilities. I am sure I can be of use somewhere and will be able to help others in their suffering….

As the woman left, she was full of energy and hope. Several months later, she told me she had recovered her health from her new task.

If we want to examine this case history scientifically, we come to the following conclusions about the connections between the somatic and psychic dimensions. It cannot be proved that her severe physical illness was in any way the consequence of her frustration and dissatisfaction with her work in the hospital. But there is hardly any doubt that her sudden improvement in her emotional state can be seen as the consequence of her perceiving a new meaning in her present situation. What we can learn from this is that we can never know exactly what part the dimension of the psyche plays in an organic (physical) illness. In contrast, we almost always may suspect a deep and genuine meaning experience behind a recovery brought about by the resources of the noëtic dimension.

The dialogue I quoted is interesting for our theme for an additional reason. The word "survival" was mentioned and had led to the question "To what end?" An answer emerged from the logotherapeutic dialogue that encouraged her to overcome her depression, an answer that made sense to many other patients in logotherapeutic treatment, namely survival for the sake of the positive possibilities that life may still have in store. No situation can be so hopeless or bungled that there are not some positive possibilities hidden in it. As long and as soon as a person is aware of this, a reason to survive exists, if only to give these possibilities a chance.

4. Survival—To What End?

Of course, such existential considerations rarely come to our minds in the hustle and bustle of everyday life, but they tend to emerge during times of illness and suffering. Almost every sick or suffering person has the wish to survive that illness or suffering. The medical or therapeutic effort is merely a tactical help to increase the chance for survival. The wish alone, however, is not enough. There is something fateful about unavoidable suffering, something that goes beyond human power. Nevertheless, it is well known that patients themselves can contribute personally toward survival of health crises. But the origin of this self-help and how it can be mobilized is less well known. Logotherapeutic research, for the first time, clarifies this question because it points out that such self-help:

1. can take place only in the noëtic dimension because it is in the physical and psychological dimension that an individual experiences illness or suffering;

2. is triggered by the forces of human resistance, especially the capacities for self-distancing and self-transcendence; and

3. requires the awareness of life potentials that makes it worthwhile to mobilize these forces for survival.

Where these three criteria are present, patients are most likely to significantly contribute to their recovery or to overcoming their suffering. But even in cases where improvement cannot be expected, as in chronic sicknesses for which no cure is available, fulfillment of the three criteria can bring some relief by making unavoidable suffering bearable—the meaning of a human life depends neither on how long nor on how pleasant it is.

SUMMARY

We started out by saying we are the only living creatures on this earth to whom nature has given the exclusively human dimension of the spirit from which we can draw the resources to resist the forces of destruction and aggression that are built into our cellular foundations. We have also considered the situation of those who are ill—especially those with psychological illnesses—and noted the parallels: Sick people, too, can and must draw from their exclusively human dimension to rise above their sufferings.

They, too, are confronted with something destructive within themselves that must be overcome through self-distancing and self-transcendence in order to free themselves for a life worth living, in spite of everything.

Seen from this perspective, the tragedy of humankind is also the tragedy of the individual: The human tragedy is how we face our fate. And fate is always incomprehensible, improbable, forever silent, the place where our anxious questions remain unanswered. Why is there so much evil in the world? Why is there so much suffering everywhere? We don't know. We don't understand. Simply put, it is not for us to pose questions, it is not we who are to question life, as Viktor Frankl realized; on the contrary, it is our task to give answers to the questions posed to us by fate. Sickness, distress, suffering, and danger are the question marks of our lives, not necessarily written by us, but to be answered by us in our own handwriting in our response to life. Everything we do or fail to do is an answer to the questions of fate.

Logotherapy maintains that explanations of human behavior by mainstream psychologists are one-sided, similar to the way psychosomatic research explains the development of symptoms. Most psychological schools tend to trace every human expression to emotional causes firmly anchored in our ancestry, childhood, or past learning processes. When we add the aspects of spirit, however, this reaction model no longer holds true because human beings do not automatically react, they respond, they show *response-ability*. And the more our answers are oriented toward a meaning, the more they liberate us from the power of an incomprehensible fate.

If we help our patients to see their anxieties, worries, and difficulties as challenges of fate to which they can find personal answers, they will find the courage to face that fate. If we let them sense some concrete possibilities in which they can fit their fate into a positive overall pattern of meaning, they will be able to master their life situation heroically. If we see the good in them, they will overcome the evil. If we show them a "what for," they will find the strength to endure everything else by themselves!

Here I return to my theme: "Survival—to what end?" Some may have been puzzled when they read that title. In this age, brimming with dangers,

4. Survival—To What End?

wouldn't it be enough to simply make sure we survive? Isn't it presumptuous, even provocative, to also ask "to what end"? Don't we first have to assure survival before we demand to know its direction?

Yes, this is true. Yet, we have reached a point where the experiences of psychotherapy are applicable on a grand scale because the behavior of humankind is alarmingly similar to a person about to commit suicide. And those considering suicide are not interested in preserving their lives on principle. Indeed, the danger of suicide can be defined as a loss of the principle of a will to live. But even when our will to live becomes dim, when our physical and psychological strength is ebbing, when the degenerative process increases, the human being can still think, and all future possibilities lie in this reflective process—in both negative and positive aspects. The negative thoughts may tempt us to resignation, but the positive demands to be heard as well.

Plants, in their peaceful manner, can survive without asking themselves "to what end"? Animals, in their aggressive manner, can also survive without posing the same question. But human beings, who must pose and answer questions originating in the exclusively noëtic dimension, cannot do this. Their aggressive inheritance—which they share with the animal kingdom and which for them has been the principle of destruction as well as the principle of survival—has come to a point where the boundaries between the two have become blurred. Life begins to destroy itself. The "*Stizostedion* fish" in human beings has begun to devour its own tail. What can stop worldwide suicide now is solely the incomprehensible counterforce of the human spirit that enables our species to accomplish incredible feats of will in direct opposition to the forces in ourselves, provided we perceive a meaning that releases the sources of energy within our spirit, a meaning that can be found in the positive possibilities of our existence to be realized.

There are many indications that this time we cannot survive with an option to ask ourselves later: "To what end?" The question must precede our survival—and may represent our only opportunity to survive. Once we know what we want to survive for, we may find the strength to bring about survival. Logotherapy, as a science, does not answer the question "what for?" but, as a meaning-oriented psychotherapy, it can guide every person who poses the question to discover the answer. In this respect, logotherapy is like the teacher of whom Kahlil Gibran wrote: "If he is indeed wise he does not bid you enter the house of his wisdom, but rather leads you to the threshold of your own mind."[1]

> What was the beginning?
>
> Bursting energy
> unfolding space and time?
>
> Hydrogen atoms
> transformed into helium?
>
> Spirals of gas
> cooling to stars?
>
> The cosmos? Light? The law?
>
> Is it truly thinkable:
> This tremendous coincidence
> out of nothing?
>
> The spirit within us
> knows without proof:
> In the beginning was Meaning!
>
> Elisabeth Lukas

---

[1] Gibran, K. (1923/1969). *The prophet.* New York: Knopf, p. 56.

CHAPTER 5

Waiting for Godot? The Logotherapeutic Alternative

According to a popular saying by Werner Sprenger, paths are made by walking them. Is this statement always true? Let us imagine a wilderness through which we make our way with difficulty. With every step forward, we create the path immediately behind us.

Nevertheless, there is a difference between this wilderness and a forest with a well-marked walking path. For wherever we are in the wilderness, there is a path *behind* us only, which we have just made. *In front of* us, there is untouched ground. If, on the other hand, we are on a walking path, there is a trail *behind* us and one *in front* of us: Behind us, the way we have already traveled; in front, the way we have yet to go. Behind us, a path that we, too, have created; in front of us, a kind of guideline which we certainly did not place there. A signpost that is there whether we follow it or not, whether we deviate from it or not; it does not force us to do anything, but merely offers orientation and direction. And, in fact, we cannot go without direction, not even in the wilderness, where we need an internal or external compass.

To be without orientation is to mark time or to travel in circles. Consequently, the quotation ought to say: "Paths are made by going in certain directions," to which we could add: "whether we are guided to them or not." This is analogous to Frankl's quote: "Meaning is the pacemaker of being," which could be slightly reworded to state: "Direction is the pacemaker of the path"—and of our path through life.¹ This is true of an entire people and of all humanity, because the direction is decisive. Quo vadis—where are you going?

To this by no means new—but burningly topical—question, there is a biblical metaphor, to which Viktor Frankl referred in his writings.² It is the story of the exodus of the people of Israel from Egypt in search of the promised land. As is well known, this arduous journey proceeded through the desert for 40 years. But the people of Israel would presumably have meandered through the desert much longer if they had not had more at their disposal than their own strength. By simply walking forward, they would certainly have created their path, but they would not have arrived in the promised land. An additional factor, a directional factor, was decisive: the *cloud*. According to biblical tradition, God's splendor moved before them in the form of a cloud, and by orienting themselves to this single cloud in the otherwise clear desert sky, the people of Israel found their way, the right way, which made arrival possible.

This analogy provides an answer to the ancient, oft-repeated question regarding where we want and ought to go in life, and offers hope that there is guidance for the human race in our time that leads to the "promised land," even if we are at a loss as to how to move forward. To decode this message—to be able to recognize *our* cloud in *our* very overcast sky—we must find criteria to make the recognition of this cloud easier. Frankl referred to three such criteria, the value of which for achieving peace and meaning I wish to elucidate.

1. The cloud is *always ahead,*
2. The cloud is *different,*
3. The cloud is *unattainable.*

---

1   Frankl, V. E. (1982). *Ärztliche Seelsorge* (10th ed.). Vienna: Deuticke, p. 78. [In English, a similar quote, "Meaning sets the pace of being" appears several times; e.g., see Frankl, V. E. (2010). *The Feeling of Meaninglessness*. Milwaukee: Marquette University Press, p. 116. –Ed.

2   Frankl, V. E. (1982). *Ärztliche Seelsorge* (10th ed.). Vienna: Deuticke.

5. Waiting for Godot? The Logotherapeutic Alternative

No cloud that fails to fulfill all of these criteria can serve as a signpost. For no such cloud would save us from the desert, as Samuel Beckett (1952) masterfully illustrated in his play *Waiting for Godot*.

1) THE CLOUD IS ALWAYS AHEAD

Let us visualize the procession of the people of Israel through the desert and imagine that the cloud does not float ahead of the walking masses, but rather hovers directly above their heads. This would have resulted in the procession coming to an abrupt halt for lack of direction. If the cloud had come closer to the people—for example, if it had descended among them—it would have enclosed them in fog and robbed them of all orientation. In other words, our path through life in small and in large matters can succeed only when something constantly hovers ahead of us. This may be an ideal, a should-condition, an individual task tailored to us—unrealized, but begging to be fulfilled. There must be something in advance of our life so that continuing to live and moving toward it has meaning.

An empirical study concluded in 1991 at the Catholic University of Lublin/Poland under the leadership of Kazimierz Popielski illustrated how this old wisdom remains valid. Popielski, a student of Frankl, used specially developed tests to investigate the so-called "noëtic temporality" of mentally healthy and mentally disturbed persons.[1] By this we understand *the period of life* with which individuals concern themselves spiritually (in the noëtic dimension), which they have in constant view. For no one can take a constant interest in his or her entire life, from the beginning to the foreseeable end. Everyone selects time periods and focuses their whole attention on them, triggering corresponding cognitive and emotional processes.

The Polish investigation of more than 300 individuals revealed that:

a) Mentally healthy people have their present and near future in view most of the time;

b) Individuals with symptoms of mental illness concern themselves mainly with their past and possibly also with the distant future.

---

1 Popielski, K. (1991). *Analiza poczucia sensu zycia. Test Noo-Dynamiki (T. N-D)* Redakcja Wydawnictw, Katolickiego Uniwersytetu Lubelskiego, Lublin.

Popielski summarized his results in this simple diagram and called the temporal characteristics of mental health *presence* and *vision*. *Presence* refers to conscious awareness of life in the present, in order not to miss its opportunities, but also directed toward the contents of a near future, which is anticipated in a *visionary way* and energetically pursued.

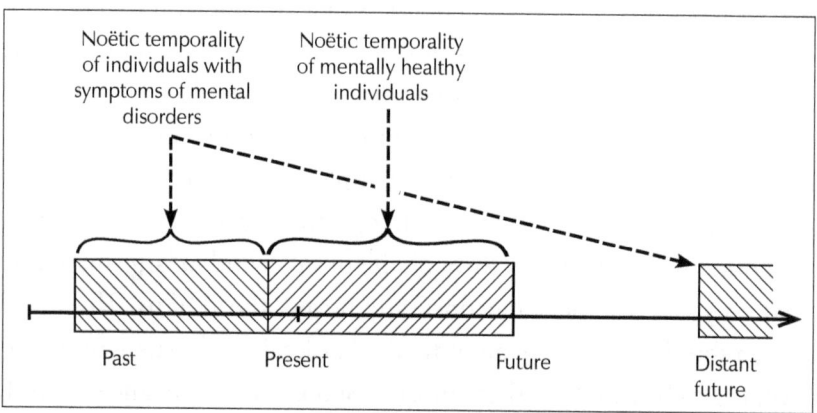

In contrast to this, it seems to be a characteristic of mental disturbances of every kind that the past and (more rarely) a scrap of the distant future are emphasized. There is certainly no harm in pausing occasionally to reflect on earlier times. Learning from the mistakes we or others have made, and feeling joy at experiences we or others have had, would be impossible without moments of remembrance. However, this looking backwards may not become, as with Lot's wife, an element of spiritual paralysis, taking control of all mental capacities of the person as usually occurs in the case of glorification of the past (in contrast to an unsatisfactory present) or condemnation of the past (as a scapegoat for all present evils). This, however, is a specific tendency of those with symptoms of mental disturbance: Either they mourn the departure of the golden days of a departed era that will never return, thus wasting present opportunities, or they declare the now-unalterable events of their past to be the necessary causes of their no less bleak and unchangeable present and tragic future—and thus become helpless victims of their biographies.

Curiously, it is the same group of people who are imprisoned by the past that also tend to be caught up in a thought world of a fantasized distant

5. Waiting for Godot? The Logotherapeutic Alternative

future, whether this be pink castles in the air of unrealistic daydreams or cataclysmic fears of an existence doomed to self-destruction. Both stances paralyze the exploitation of present resources for the pursuit of realistically attainable and ethically responsible goals just as happens with an obsession with the past.

We have said that those with symptoms of mental disturbance have these tendencies. Perhaps the converse statement cannot be rejected either, namely that people whose noëtic temporality focuses on the past and distant future suffer disturbances so that they fail to reach the promised land because they lose sight of the cloud. What would have become of the people of Israel if they had constantly looked over their shoulders in the desert in insatiable longing for the lush gardens on the banks of the Nile or shook their fists in impotent rage at the Egyptian villains who had inexorably forced their exodus? Or what would have become of them if they had blindly stumbled along, losing themselves in illusionary fantasies of the promised land which no one had yet seen, or had given in to the despair of an apparently certain death, which was anything but certain?

It is surely not far-fetched to symbolize the period of life corresponding to the "noëtic temporality" of mentally healthy people by the segment of the path between the people of Israel and the shadow of the guiding cloud.

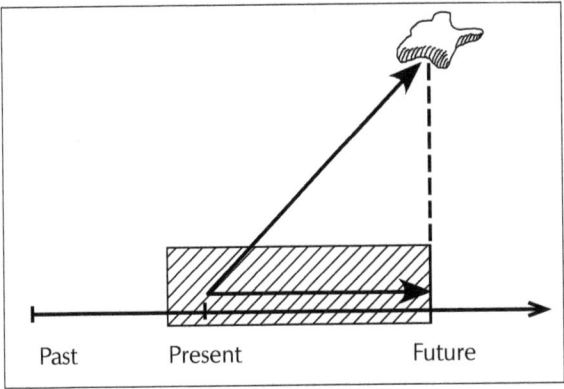

Which means that we, too, after careful exploration of our present location—the doctrines of depth psychology notwithstanding—should look ahead, but not too far, only to the point where the "call of meaning"

(Frankl) can still be heard, summoning us to meaningful action, to the next step. Look ahead in the knowledge that there is something that is always in advance of us and never leaves us. Only in this way is peace with the past and constructive change of the present toward a promising future possible.

2) THE CLOUD IS DIFFERENT

The biblical story tells us something more: The cloud is essentially different from the people following it. It is of a different quality, "of higher value," superior. It was not members of the people of Israel who led the people through the desert, not leaders, advance scouts, gurus, people in power, or people of flesh and blood. The cloud glided, so to speak, on a level of being higher than that of those who entrusted themselves to it.

Once again, we can ask whether the converse holds: Do only those who entrust themselves to a "higher reality" on their path through life find their way into the promised land? How many people have erred, only because they followed false idols, or were blinded by false promises? How many fearful, timid people have oriented themselves by the opinions of their peers, wishing to do right by their colleagues and supervisors at any price and being led to do stupid things? How many immature adolescents and young adults sell themselves body and soul to their peer group, commit criminal acts under pressure, or voluntarily surrender to the clutches of a cult? How many uncritical followers surround politicians, actors, sports stars, and financial bosses, whose rise and fall result from only money and prestige?

It is the question of the scale against which the direction of a path through life is measured, a question that cannot be answered on the same plane on which it is asked. No person can tell others where they have to go, where their promised land might lie. We are not the paradigm—neither for ourselves nor for our fellow human beings—but nevertheless the paradigm *is within us*. Frankl identified it as our *personal conscience*, a concept which he clearly separated from the Freudian concept of the superego, by which the sum of learned norms and accepted moral laws is meant. In contrast,

5. Waiting for Godot? The Logotherapeutic Alternative

the personal conscience "heeds the voice of transcendence";[1] it is—in terms of the biblical metaphor—the finger pointing to the cloud.

In this context, let us mention the work of Hans Küng, titled "Project World Ethos."[2] Here he illustrated why an undivided world needs an undivided ethos:

> What use are new laws to individual states and organizations, whether the EEC [now the EU –Ed], the USA, or the UN, when a majority of humanity have no intention of adhering to them and constantly find ways and means of irresponsibly asserting personal or collective interests? (p. 56)

As an example, he added

> In the next five years, new prison cells will have to be built in the USA for 460,000 new prisoners at a cost of 35 billion dollars because of the new wave of drug abuse. For economic reasons alone, the demand for more control, police, jails, and stricter laws cannot be the only solution to overcome such serious problems of our time. (p. 57)

The relevance of these arguments can be seen in the various areas of unrest on this earth, to which resolutions of the World Security Council or cease-fire agreements cannot bring peace, any more than the threat of a military strike to end the conflict violently. Also of little use in reducing inhumanity and brutality on our earth are analyses of causes. Looking to the past to discover cultural and political causes of present miseries does not automatically end them, which is not surprising, given that "the cloud is always ahead." More essential for constructive change than any knowledge of the negative causes is the recognition of *reasons for the positive*. In his reflections, Küng (1992) seized upon this old logotherapeutic rule:

> Why should a criminal not kill his hostages, a dictator not rape his people, a business group not exploit its country, a nation not begin a war, a power block not fire missiles at the

---

1 Frankl, V. E. (1991). *Der Wille zum Sinn* Munich: Piper, p. 117.

2 Küng, H. (1992). *Projekt Weltethos (4th ed.)*. Munich: Piper.

other half of humanity, if this lies in their deepest personal interest? (p. 76)

What, then, are genuine reasons for positive actions? That fear of punishment does not suffice has long been clear. Could it be purely rational reasons, survival strategies, logical deductions from Kant's "categorical imperative"? The generally observable discrepancy between the present intelligence of human beings and their moral behavior gives rise to strong doubts, which led Küng (1992) to point to another level:

> No, the categorical of the ethical claim, the unconditionality of "ought to," can be founded not by the human being, the multiply conditional human being, but rather only by something unconditional; by an absolute which is capable of imparting an all-encompassing meaning and which includes and permeates the individual human being, also human nature, even the entire human community. That can be only the last, highest reality itself which, although it is not rationally proven can be accepted in reasonable trust—however this is called, understood, and interpreted in the different religions. (p. 77)

Is this not a reference to the cloud in its "differentness"? Küng reached the conclusion that human beings cannot truly live together without a world ethos of nations, and that there can be no peace between nations without peace between religions because only the *shared insights* of the various religions with their binding character could unite those participating in them. He is right. Only when what is good for the one is no longer bad for the other, and vice versa; e.g., what is good for an economic group is no longer bad for their country—only when a concept of the good and meaningful emerges, which is *unconditionally good* and to which both sides agree, will human beings live together in consensus and peace.

Such an unconditional good is no longer the subject of diplomatic negotiations, which must attempt to mediate between contradictory interests, but rather the subject of the one overriding human concern, which peaks in the search for the promised land. It is endlessly different from everything that appears useful, advantageous, and profitable in the experience of us

5. Waiting for Godot? The Logotherapeutic Alternative

earthlings, conditioned as it is by a great variety of factors. For Frankl, it was the voice of transcendence, audible in the personal conscience. For Küng, it was the world ethos, readable in the overlapping basic substance of the world religions. We will certainly not err if we call the latter the collective manifestation of the former.

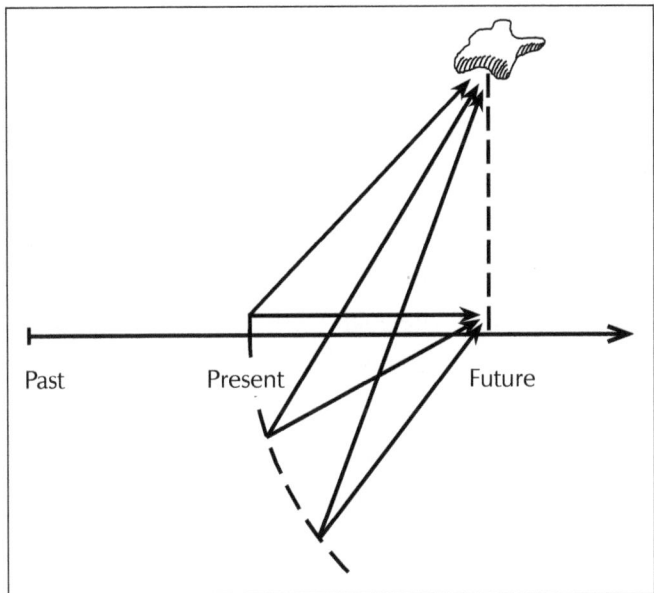

It would be advisable for us to concur in this "thought pattern" of hope, for in the desert there is no other hope. But why should humanity not set out together on some distant day, when the pain has become great enough, as once did the people of Israel, setting out from various locations, but united in a common view of a higher reality?

3. THE CLOUD IS UNATTAINABLE

For those individuals who have already set out to follow the cloud, what do we learn in the biblical metaphor about what happens to them? The answer is twofold:

The first lesson from the biblical metaphor is that none of them arrives at the cloud. This statement may seem strange, but it is worth spending a little time on it. Obviously, it is meaningful during our journey through life to strive for the unattainable; in other words, to aim for the optimum in order to achieve the maximum that is within our own limitations. Opposed to this is the view, widespread in psychology, that one should pursue smaller, moderate goals within easy reach (which correspond to available reserves of strength), rather than making lofty plans (which demand too much). Overambitious plans produce only disappointment and feelings of failure.

The contradiction is apparent, because no member of the people of Israel intended during the 40-year journey to arrive at the cloud. The small, moderate goal of every one of them was always the next fixed point in the sand and rock beneath the cloud, where its shadow fell. But these fixed points could not have been found were it not for the reference point in the sky.

Generalizing, it can be observed that people who are plagued by disappointments and feelings of failure often confuse the reference point with the fixed points. For them, the goal is both, and reaching both "goals" is necessary for happiness—an impossibility!

An example: A mother wants the best for her child. She spends time informing herself about raising children; she plays and exercises with her child. But at school, her child's performance leaves a lot to be desired. He is forced to transfer to a less demanding school, meets friends who persuade him to skip classes, receives poor final grades and drops out of an apprenticeship after a few weeks. He has become one of those unemployed young adults who hang around on the streets and get by on occasional jobs. His mother is desperate and deeply disappointed.

What is the reference source in this example, the unattainable cloud? The mother's love wishes for the complete good of the child, for total success in life; this is legitimate, for love sees the beloved in the fullness of his human worth, almost "as God intended him."[1] From this reference source, all fixed points can be derived in the form of small, moderate tasks that the mother discovers from birth as "assigned" to her, e.g. nursing the child, supporting the child in toilet training, getting the child acclimated to kindergarten. Every successive fixed point is a step in the right direction, one not only suited to the ability of the mother, but also in the realm of possibility. Even

---

[1] Frankl, V. E. (1982). *Ärztliche Seelsorge* (10th ed.). Vienna: Deuticke, p. 146. [In English, "...the way God 'meant' him" is on p. 149, *The doctor and the soul* –Ed.]

5. Waiting for Godot? The Logotherapeutic Alternative

in the present unemployment of her son a new fixed point is apparent on the mother's path, whether it consists of not allowing dialogue to end, performing an act of trust, or giving concrete help.

If the mother accepted her child as he is, and at the same time remained constantly on her own path from one fixed point to the next, she would have a good chance of reaching the "promised land," where love is stronger than need or death. However, if she wants her son to change, if she fanatically seeks to bring about his good, if she desperately searches for explanations of his "failure," if she believes that she has done everything wrong in his upbringing; in short, if she cannot accept the stony paths of life and clings to internal protest, then despair will result. For the cloud which floats ahead of her is unattainable.

The second lesson from the biblical metaphor is that we learn that most of the people of Israel who left Egypt never reached the "promised land," but that it was rather their children or grandchildren who finally reached the destination of the journey. According to this, it can be important to sow seeds, although later generations will harvest the fruits. And some trailblazing finds its meaning in allowing others to reach the destination.

Moreover, we do not know with which metaphysical framework to interpret the story. Could it not be possible that those who faithfully followed the cloud and died in the desert reached the "promised land" before their comrades who survived them? Yes, is it not thinkable, that the actual promised land begins beyond time and space and there, the arrival on the cloud, which in our world is never possible, is no longer Utopian, but a true gift of grace?

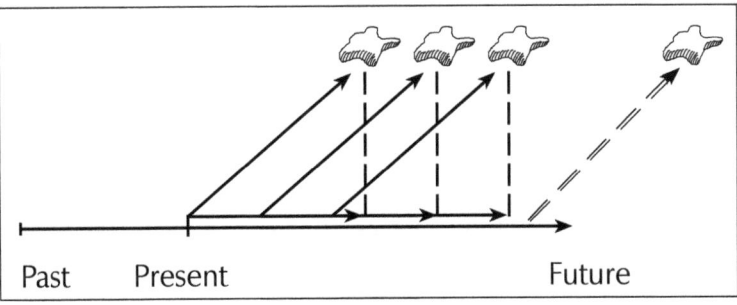

In any case, the country into which the people of Israel were led has hitherto so little deserved the title "promised land" that it seems safe to assume that the promise of the cloud found and finds its fulfillment on a plane not comprehensible to us nor accessible in words.

After thus discussing criteria that can give an up-to-date answer to the question "Quo vadis?," we want to visit in our imagination the (supposedly) *cloudless desert*. As mentioned, this is well illustrated in the drama *Waiting for Godot*. Here, there is no ideal in advance of the given situation. Although Mr. Godot is expected to say what should be done, he belongs to the category "people like you and me"—a deceptive expectation. And striving for the unattainable is rejected out of hand as senseless with the result that the unattainable slips away. In this desert, one cannot live or die. Since our human society is at present flirting dangerously with the status of "waiting for Godot," Beckett's warning should be briefly recapitulated.

The drama begins with the representation of the actual situation of the human world, embodied by two figures, Vladimir and Estragon. Suffering and fear prevail.

Vladimir: No one ever suffers but you. I don't count…

ങ

Estragon: Who am I to tell my private nightmares to if I can't tell them to you?

What are they suffering from? Lack of orientation, unwillingness to take initiative, lack of a sense of responsibility, hopelessness. In Frankl's terminology, an existential vacuum. From a lowered gaze, in the biblical metaphor, to which only sand and no cloud is revealed.

Vladimir: Let's wait and see what he says.
Estragon: Who?
Vladimir: Godot.
Estragon: Good idea.
Vladimir: Let's wait till we know exactly how we stand.

ങ

5. Waiting for Godot? The Logotherapeutic Alternative

Vladimir: Nothing you can do about it.

Estragon: No use struggling.

Vladimir: One is what one is.

Estragon: No use wriggling.

Vladimir: The essential doesn't change.

But the meaning void of this world is only apparent. A call of meaning sounds. It appears in the form of Pozzo and Lucky, as master and slave, as oppressed and oppressor, as injustice crying out to be overcome. There is a rope around Lucky's neck with which Pozzo commands him. The two representatives of the human world see quite clearly what is happening but they are lost in lethargy and resignation.

Vladimir: Look!

Estragon: What?

Vladimir (pointing): His neck.

☙

Estragon: Oh I say!

Vladimir: A running sore.

Estragon: It's the rope.

Vladimir: It's the rubbing.

Estragon: It's inevitable.

Vladimir: It's the knot.

Estragon: It's the chafing.

☙

Vladimir: It's inevitable.

☙

Suddenly, in the middle of their foolishness, their personal conscience is moved, hearing the "call of meaning," and for a moment the two recognize the cloud which shows them the way.

Vladimir (crying out): It's a scandal!

❦

Pozzo (to Vladimir): Are you alluding to anything in particular?

Vladimir (stutteringly resolute): To treat a man… (gesture toward Lucky)… like that… I think that… no… a human being… no… it's a scandal!

Estragon (not to be outdone): A disgrace!

❦

The master diverts them skillfully:

Pozzo: Think twice now before you do anything rash.… What happens in this case to your appointment with this… Godot?

❦

The master soothes them with excuses and distortions of the facts.

Pozzo: …instead of driving him away as I might have done, I mean instead of simply kicking him out on his arse, in the goodness of my heart I am bringing him to the fair, where I hope to get a good price for him.

❦

Lucky's crying proves him a liar, but the master uses the trick of hypocrisy.

Pozzo: Comfort him, since you pity him.

❦

He knows in advance how a feeble attempt to comfort the tormented creature will end. In his pain, Lucky lashes out and the two representatives of the human world are "cured" of their fit of pity. All ridicule of Lucky that follows fails to move their hearts, so that the call of meaning echoes unheeded in the desert. Vladimir and Estragon do not understand that Godot has shown himself to them in their neighbor. They are waiting for a Godot on the same level on which they stand. They listen to the false prophet who visits them in the form of a seemingly harmless boy.

Boy: Mr. Godot told me to tell you he won't come this evening but surely tomorrow.

5. Waiting for Godot? The Logotherapeutic Alternative

How could they have recognized the false prophet? By one fact about Mr. Godot.

Vladimir: Is he good to you?

Boy: Yes.

Vladimir: He doesn't beat you?

Boy: No sir, not me.

Vladimir: Whom does he beat?

Boy: He beats my brother, sir.

To wait for a Mr. Godot who strikes is ridiculous—the punitive image of God is a self-contradiction. Somehow, the two representatives of the human race sense this.

Vladimir: We've nothing more to do here.

☙

Estragon: Well, shall we go?

Vladimir: Yes, let's go.

☙

They do not go, however, and thus the drama continues in the second act, which begins with a sprouting tree. Nature and life offer their powers of renewal. However, Vladimir and Estragon are not receptive to this because they are oriented to the past and not to the future.

> Estragon: All my lousy life I've crawled about in the mud! And you talk to me about scenery! (Looking wildly about him) Just look at this muck-heap! I've never stirred from it!

☙

According to the noëtic temporality of the mentally ill, they are obsessed not only with the past, but also fall victim to "castles in the air."

Vladimir: That is Godot! At last!... We're saved!

☙

Estragon: I'm accursed!

Vladimir: Were you far off?

Estragon: To the edge of the cliff... I lost my head.

☙

The two representatives of the human world begin to notice that they are at the edge of the cliff, of the chasm. Horrified, they turn their searching gaze skyward.

Estragon: Do you think God sees me?... God have pity on me!

Vladimir (vexed): And me?

Estragon: On me! On me! Pity! On me!

☙

Pity arrives immediately in the form of a new chance for humanity and human dignity, in the form of an impressive lesson, and in the form of a return signal: If you want mercy, practice mercy! All this is expressed in Pozzo and Lucky, who once again enter the scene as emissaries of the cloud. But this time not as oppressor and oppressed, but rather as the double opportunity of practicing mercy: consolation of the innocent and forgiveness of the guilty. Pozzo, the powerful, blinded by his own cruelty, has fallen, and Lucky has also collapsed under his burden.

Pozzo: Here! Here! Help me up!

Vladimir: He can't get up... Perhaps he has another bone for you.

Estragon: Bone?

Vladimir: Chicken. Do you not remember?

☙

Estragon: We should ask for the bones first? Then if he refuses we'll leave him here.

Vladimir: You mean we have him at our mercy?

Estragon: Yes.

Vladimir: And that we should subordinate our good offices to certain conditions?

5. Waiting for Godot? The Logotherapeutic Alternative

Estragon: What?

Vladimir: That seems intelligent all right.

⁂

At this point, the two representatives of the human world lose their footing and begin figuratively to slide down the cliff face toward the chasm.

Pozzo: Help, I'll pay you!

Estragon: How much?

Pozzo: One hundred francs!

Estragon: It's not enough.

⁂

Pozzo: Two hundred!

Vladimir: We wait. We are bored… We are bored to death.

⁂

Pozzo: Pity! Pity!

⁂

Estragon: Make him stop it. Kick him in the crotch.

Vladimir (striking Pozzo): Will you stop it! Crablouse!

⁂

The representatives of the human world depart from the "world ethos."

Estragon: Look at the little cloud.

Vladimir (raising his eyes): Where?

Estragon: There. In the zenith.

Vladimir: Well? What is there so wonderful about it? [Silence]

Estragon: Let's pass on to something else, do you mind.

Vladimir: I was just going to suggest it.

Estragon: But to what?

⁂

The "something else" consists of brutally kicking the innocent Lucky, thus banishing any chance of humanity from their existence. Pozzo and Lucky withdraw. The wait for Godot remains, the wait for the "man with the white beard" whose coming has been announced by the boy and who should tell them what to do.

However, love can be practiced only voluntarily without calculation; if it is purchased or dictated, its nature is corrupted. If it were ordered from above, obedience would no longer be love. Before one walks the way to the "promised land," it *must be chosen voluntarily with honest motives.*

Estragon and Vladimir did not choose it, and thus they are left standing at the tree which was sprouting new leaves at the beginning of the second act, now trying to find a way of hanging themselves from its naked branches.

Estragon: You haven't got a bit of rope?

Vladimir: No.

༄

Estragon: Wait, there's my belt.

Vladimir: It's too short.

Estragon: You could hang on to my legs.

Vladimir: And who'd hang on to mine?

Estragon: True.

༄

In the (supposedly) *cloudless desert,* life is symbolized by the fresh leaves of the tree, and death is symbolized by its withered branches, but they do not succeed. With this central statement, the curtain falls on Beckett's play. The curtain of the theatre of the world, on whose stage the real human race appears, has not fallen yet; the third act (the third millennium after Christ) is about to begin.

Will we, the actors, understand before it is too late—before we literally wrap a rope around our necks—that "Godot" (the cloud, the call of meaning, love and mercy) is *waiting for us*?

5. Waiting for Godot? The Logotherapeutic Alternative

Frankl (1947) ended his book *Existenzanalyse und die Probleme der Zeit* with the prophetic words:

> If it is true that human beings are like actors on a stage, then let us remember that the actor—blinded by the lights—sees a black hole instead of the audience. He never sees in front of whom he is acting. And is it not similar for the human being? He is blinded by the light of daily life and does not see to whom he has responsibility for his existence (just as the actor is responsible for his role): He does not see who he is acting for. Nevertheless, there are always people who think: Just where we think we see nothing, the Great Spectator sits and watches us relentlessly. These are the people who call out to us: Be careful—you're standing in front of the open curtain![1]

Let us consider his words not merely as *the* logotherapeutic answer to Estragon's question: "Do you think God sees me?," but rather as *the* appropriate motto for the beginning of the third act in the theatre of life in which everything is still possible: arrival and downfall.

---

1 Cited in Frankl, V. E. (1991). *Der Wille zum Sinn* (new ed.). Munich: Piper, p. 107. [In English, see Frankl, V. E. (1988). *The will to meaning.* New York: Penguin, pp. 152-153.]

The condition of earth
is critical;
there are many indications
of a terrible catastrophe.

The condition of animals
is critical;
many fight in vain for survival
in a terrible existence.

The condition of forests
is critical;
many show visible signs
of a terrible destruction.

The condition of humankind
is critical;
many sense the warning
of a terrible responsibility.

The condition of terror, however,
is not critical,
but an incentive
to meaningful action—now!

Elisabeth Lukas

CHAPTER 6

From Self-Actualization to Global Responsibility: Search for the Sacred, the Necessary, and Otherliness

I would like to begin with a personal childhood recollection. I was born during the war. My grandparent's house was bombed and therefore they had to live with my parents in our two-room apartment. In the years just after the war, my grandparents sometimes had an argument that amused my parents. It was no marital tiff—my grandparents were devoted to each other. But curiously, it was just that devotion that spawned the argument. The argument was triggered by a cup of coffee left over from breakfast and saved for an afternoon warm-up. The following dialogue ensued:

Grandfather: "Here, have this cup of coffee, it will be good for you."

Grandmother: [Promptly] "No, no, *you* have it. I'm not thirsty."

Grandfather: [Insistently] "Take it. You need it more than I do."

Grandmother: "I'm fine. You'd really be doing me a favor to drink it."

And so they played that game until the coffee got cold. Each urged the other, knowing that the dose of caffeine (if it were there at all) would give the undernourished body of the other strength to hold out until the evening.

Yet, all this happened in my grandparents' generation, at a time in which psychology stressed the concept: "Think of yourself, give yourself a treat." And indeed, this psychology was partially correct, because it tended to protect people from their mania for making sacrifices.

Now let us return to our time. Recently, I counseled the parents of a one-year-old and a three-year-old. The parental conflict was about how to plan their vacations. The mother said to the father: "I've had the kids for the whole year. Now I want to recuperate for at least three weeks. That's why I want you to take care of them and let me go on vacation." "No way," answered the father. "I work all year for the family, and when I'm on vacation I want to relax without noisy kids."

"You never think of *me*," shouted the mother. "If you saddle me with them, how can I ever get a rest?" "I don't care," shrugged the father, "but I'm not going to take them."

As I listened, I pictured them as two tired, aging individuals in the postwar years, arguing in a poorly furnished kitchen over a cup of coffee, each trying to snatch it from the other....

Times have changed; a new generation has grown up. I do not claim that this feuding couple is typical of the present generation but it must be recognized that the desire to make sacrifices has become rare. What happens when psychology repeatedly peddles its old ego-centered platitudes—when all it has to offer the vacation-hungry couple is that they should think of themselves? Don't we need a different mantra today? Isn't it the obligation of psychologists and psychotherapists to balance unhealthy extremes? And don't these scientists have to ask themselves just *which* extremes cause the worse disturbances?

Our history looks back at a long, dark period when individuals enslaved by various stresses had trouble self-actualizing themselves, as we call it. This period is about to end. An even darker period is dawning, in which our world is enslaved by many stresses—stresses triggered by our economic pressures, social media, overpopulation and technology. Self-actualization of individuals is no longer a primary need. We need a widespread acknowledgement of each individual's responsibility within the population, an awareness that we are co-responsible for what goes on in the world. The

6. From Self-Actualization to Global Responsibility

meaningless mania for making sacrifices must be replaced by something new, namely a meaningful readiness for making sacrifices in the name of the world community. Self-centeredness is no longer an acceptable alternative.

Among the serious contemporary psychological movements, logotherapy is the one that never advocated egoism. Its basic idea is *education toward responsibility*, a concept formulated when occupation with the human psyche was still considered mere "navel contemplation," albeit navel contemplation through precise psychotherapeutic lenses. The logotherapist maintains that only understanding our individual psychodynamic nature is not sufficient to enable us to conduct our lives in a way fitting to human nature.

The human being is by nature a spiritual, noëtic being, and hence in our spiritual search we reach out for the suprahuman. Human contemplation cannot stop at the navel; it reaches further along the umbilical cord for the "whence" of life, the "whereto" of life and, thus, the meaning of life.

For this search, psychotherapeutic lenses are not enough; we also must use philosophical and theological lenses and even these do not reveal the suprahuman dimension—we can only glimpse a reflection of it. Logotherapy calls this reflection the *meaning of the moment* or the *demand of the situation*, postulating that each moment of human existence has a particular meaningfulness that can be discovered and met. When this happens, this moment or situation is in harmony with that unfathomable suprahuman dimension that contains ultimate meaning.

Let me cite a simple example. Last winter, I went by train to give a seminar in a city in the north of Germany. The seminar was successful and I was presented with a beautiful bouquet of flowers. Orchids and suitcase in hand, I battled my way in the wintry cold to the railroad station, wondering what to do with the flowers. If I took them in the heated train compartment to Munich, nine hours away, they would wilt.

The easiest solution would have been to discard them in a trash can at the station. But it seemed a waste of these fine flowers chosen with such loving care. I could not bring myself to throw them away and took them with me on the train.

As expected, it was very warm in the compartment and I opened the window. At the end of the platform I saw a woman leaning on a railing, shoulders drooping. She seemed tired and saddened, as if weighted down by sorrow. Now I suddenly knew the meaning of the moment. I ran out of the train and, flowers in hand, addressed the woman: "Excuse me, may I give you these flowers? I am on my way to Munich and I don't expect them to survive the long trip."

The woman raised her careworn face. "It's been a long time since anybody gave me flowers," she answered quietly. As I rushed to the train I had just enough time to call back: "Well, then it's about time that somebody did it!" As the train pulled out of the station, I stood by the window and saw her waving to me and smiling.

Yes, the incident was trifling. Or was it something more? It could as well have been a peak experience for a lonely human being. I am not citing the episode for its possible effect on the woman, but to highlight the unique meaning of a unique situation: to give those flowers, which would have perished, to a person to whom they brought joy.

Among all my alternatives there was just this one meaningful possibility. If I had not recognized it or had let it pass, it would have been wasted. On the other hand, in making the possibility a reality, it did not pass by but passed into reality where it may find its place in ultimate meaning.

To generalize, one might say that logotherapy, like any other psychotherapy, tries to bring to consciousness what in a critical situation may not be conscious. But we are not talking here about making people aware of repressed traumas or secret desires. We are talking about making people aware of 1) *alternatives available* at a given time; 2) *meaningful possibilities among the alternatives available* at a given time; 3) *their responsibility for realizing those meaningful possibilities* among the alternatives available at a given time.

If these three steps are taken, individuals are able to do something good in this world. And those who do good in the world do the best for themselves, although this may not have been their primary intention.

6. From Self-Actualization to Global Responsibility

This may sound very rational, but becoming aware of something is not in itself a rational act. We become consciously aware of something only when, beyond understanding, we deeply *feel* what is important at that moment. Reason and feeling participate equally in making us aware; intellect must team up with emotional vibrations in transmuting blindness into insight. We recognize meaning when it touches us, but to act upon that meaning we, of course, have to allow the meaning to touch us. Thus logotherapy is not only concerned with rational considerations, as some critics say, but also with the stimulation and actualization of feelings.

However, in stimulating and actualizing feelings we must be careful not to become "feeling exhibitionists," which are so popular in Western psychological culture. In contrast to Asian cultures, in which a show of feeling is taboo and it is thus a virtue to hide one's feelings, in our culture it has become a fad to publicly uncover one's feelings. This open display of feelings may well be the result of that navel contemplation mentioned earlier. It is evident that people—trained in self-actualization and self-experience—begin to see nothing but their own navels and tend to consider nothing to be more important than navel exposition.

Nor is this all. Feelings that well up during such self-inspections are usually detached from the real, outside world. They amount to petty fears, narcissistic desires, strong frustrations, and plaintive self-pitying, which serve no creative purpose and result in a river of endless complaints about life's burdens. In that river, the power station of responsibility has no place; its flow yields no energy potential. The world cannot be saved by people who make their own psychic condition the focus of their lives and are oblivious to the extrapsychic reality around them.

More is at stake in today's world than taking care of some psychological discomfort, and we have more to gain than merely our own inner equilibrium! We must be concerned about a *future worthy of human beings*, for us and for our children. This concern deserves the trouble it takes to look up from our navels and focus our feeling on something beyond our egotistic feelings, which in turn could release energies for the spiritual renewal of our generation.

Logotherapy points to three areas of sensitivity which we ought to reactivate in order to become more receptive to the meaning of the moment and to be more ready for the demand of the situation. These sensitivities are:

1) the feeling for the Sacred,

2) the feeling for the Necessary,

3) the feeling for Otherliness.

The following comments on these sensitivities are designed to pave the way from self-actualization toward global responsibility, or simply from I to You, to We, and to Him.

THE FEELING FOR THE SACRED

What is meant by the Sacred? In becoming human, we have righted ourselves, as it were, and now extend in two directions: "up" toward Transcendence and "down" to Nature. With our foreheads we reach into infinity above, while our feet are firmly planted on earth. The two directions symbolize our ties to our biological and biochemical roots and to our spiritual home as expressed in the Latin term *religare*, to tie back.

Both ties have loosened, to our disadvantage. In my travels through South America last year, I was shocked by the widespread poverty. But I was particularly struck by the fact that the miserable slums at the periphery of the big cities are surrounded by large areas of untilled land, where several harvests of fruit and vegetables could easily be raised each year. I was told that even farmers who own land often let it lie fallow and move to the big cities where they expect a more comfortable life; instead, however, they decline morally and economically.

I am well aware that the complex problems of Third World countries defy a common denominator. Yet, if such a denominator of their problems were to be found, it would probably be the loss of a healthy tie to the Sacred: Nature and her treasures.

Such a common denominator would also apply to industrialized nations, as demonstrated by emerging environmental problems. Yet there are indications that we suffer even more from our waning relationship

6. From Self-Actualization to Global Responsibility

to Transcendence. Indeed, a revitalized wave of mysticism happens to be passing over us at present, but much of it is superficial, far from the essential. Therefore it is important to rediscover the feeling for the essential, for true wonder, for that which is big in small things, for what is valuable in what seems worthless—in short, the feeling for the Sacred.

Take an older adult with symptoms of advanced dementia, for example. He lies in bed, motionless with a blank expression on his face. What does this mean? It means that his spiritual self is unable to manifest itself and that we, too, are unable to get through to him. But the spiritual self of this human being exists undamaged and exists beyond the possibility of being damaged. It is only obscured by a worn-out body and confers on it its human dignity. The same is true of a newborn baby. The baby, too, can be called "blank," and also carries a spiritual potential which makes the baby unique. For that reason, a baby deserves the love and respect of the parents, even as the old man deserves the love and respect of his children. Viktor Frankl convincingly demonstrated this in his writings.

Let us think of the grail. We see only the bowl. What it represents, its inner essence, is concealed. We bow our heads because the bowl carries a holy content. Now let us think of an apple seed. A sliver of wood. Yet inside is the potential for a large, strong, many-branched tree. Think of a fertilized egg. A spot of phlegm. But what abundance of life it carries! Take a normal cell of a human being or an animal—a little glob of amino acid. Yet what richness of genetic information it contains! Or a rock, which is merely some inorganic material. Each atom is part of an artwork of order, motion, and electric charge! We have to relearn to look behind the outer shell: into the interior, into the core of matter, or into the core of a person where creation pulsates; we will never cease to be amazed.

The miracle is in the potential of being. Each single, invisible atom has the potential of a tiny nuclear bomb. Each single, invisible cell protects and harbors the potential of a living being. Each single human body is the potential home of spirituality, freedom, and responsibility. The blank face, the apple seed, the rock are on par with the grail. They contain the unfathomable, revealed to those who can see, although even they cannot see beyond the grail's rim. What's inside is beyond the human capacity to understand.

If we thus expand our feeling for the Sacred, we can restore our relationship to Transcendence and to Nature. This would be beneficial to ourselves, as well as to our fellow human beings and to the environment. Who would act in a meaningless way, if he or she firmly believed that even the most miserable human being had dignity and the most trivial object value? We would not casually destroy Nature if we saw in it our own roots.

Nor would we deny an ultimate meaning, if we spiritually felt at home in it. If we practice reverence and sensitivity in our relations with everything that exists, we will experience a new tie with all Being.

THE FEELING FOR THE NECESSARY

To make a point here, I have to resort to a linguistic crutch. The German word for "necessary" or "needful" is *notwendig*. Literally translated, the first part of the word means "need" in the sense of misery, and the second part of the word means "turning around" in the sense of alleviating the misery. Therefore if something is necessary ("not wendig") it means that some need or misery has to be turned around or alleviated.

That brings us to the feeling for "that which is necessary." Frankl defines the meaning of the moment as "that for which a need exists" or "that which matters." To find that meaning, we have to focus on what is essential, on that which turns the need around and improves what has to be improved, and what turns a negative into a positive or completes an incomplete.

Now, it is a sociological phenomenon that, as civilization progresses, the obvious necessities recede into the background. In earlier times, when a parent worked all day for a farmer in the fields and still had housework to do and five children to raise, there was always something waiting in the wings that needed to be done to turn around a need—field work, housework, or caring for children. Finding meaning was no problem.

6. From Self-Actualization to Global Responsibility

Today, in contrast, when a parent works a few hours a week, has the usual household gadgets, and cares for one child (who is in school or in child care all day), there is more free time: nothing that "needs turning," nothing to be done. In this situation, when the obvious needs to satisfy the routine daily requirements are reduced, the question of meaning asserts itself.

However, the newly won freedom results in a peculiar polarization. Some people use their freedom with joy and a wealth of ideas: They start a garden, attend lectures, do volunteer work, read books, cultivate friendships, or go on trips. Others get lost in their new freedom, sink into passivity and apathy, and experience a spiritual emptiness that eventually, when it becomes unbearable, is filled with watching television, overeating, or drug addiction. The question is: At what point does it come to this divide? When does a person tend to use freedom meaningfully or not?

Giselher Guttmann, the director of the Psychological Institute at the University of Vienna, has given us important insights into this problem. He discovered, through ergopsychometric measurements, that in challenging situations some people mobilize additional forces that stimulate their work, whereas others fail, although under neutral conditions the "failures" perform just as well as the first group. For example, runners attaining the same speeds in training fall into two groups: those who in the challenge of the race are slower than they otherwise are—facetiously referred to as "training champs"—and those who in the actual race achieve more than their usual speed and often emerge victorious.

It is no mystery. We know why people with the same abilities exhibit such different levels of achievement when it comes to the test. It depends on *what they think in critical situations*: whether they think about themselves or are oblivious of themselves. If they think of themselves, they are gripped by fear; fear of making fools of themselves, of disappointing friends, of being at the mercy of a hostile fate. People who primarily think of themselves in critical situations invariably fear the consequences of failure. Such *anticipatory anxiety*, as Frankl called it, activates the cerebral cortex, in fact overactivates it, leading to failure. In this way emotional factors block spiritual capabilities.

The situation is different for people concentrating on the challenge of the moment and not thinking of themselves. They focus on the task before them and harness their resources as best they can. The stress of having to prove themselves does not block them but triggers maximum concentration, which again is reflected in the cerebral cortex. This maximal focus creates optimal capacity for achievement.

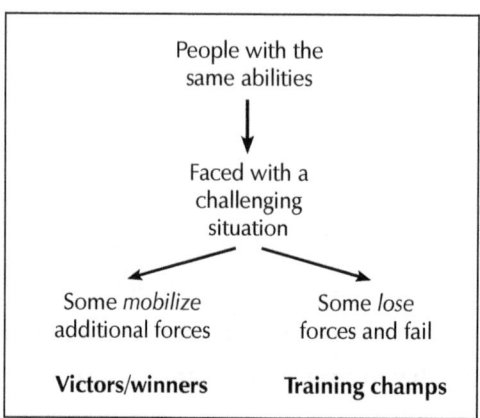

Two conclusions follow: First, intelligence and aptitude tests, normally conducted in stress-free situations, tell nothing about the candidate's conduct in actual life situations; this consideration offers a serious reason for psychologists to revise their traditional testing methods. Second, the reason for failure under stress often is not overstraining, as has been thought, but rather self-induced egocentric fear. And this is a reason to revise the traditional stress theory. But these two conclusions need not concern us because I have something else in mind. I want to apply Guttmann's findings to the phenomenon mentioned earlier: Some people use their free time meaningfully and some don't.

The parallel seems clear. Those who get trapped in a meaning crisis when freed from previously necessary work, and spend their days in dull passivity and pathological emptiness, are comparable to the training champs. The others, who when liberated blossom into creativity, are the victors. In short, what looks like a release from the prison of work is in truth a challenging situation, a time of "existential probation."

6. From Self-Actualization to Global Responsibility

As long as circumstances dictate, and we are obliged to do this or that, we act as we are told—life gives the orders. To reintroduce the example of the woman who works for the farmer: When children are hungry, they must be fed; when laundry gets soiled, it must be washed; when cows' udders are full, they must be milked. The woman fulfills her obligations well or poorly, willingly or not, but apart from that she has little choice.

However, as soon as free time opens up and the dictates of the situation abate, we must choose our activities and we are responsible for our choice. That puts us on probation. Now *we*, not life, decide what we do with our talent, our knowledge, our unstructured hours, our money and power. *We* determine how we spend our material and spiritual capital.

But—most importantly—it would be wrong to believe that in this situation necessities cease to exist. They do exist, although they are no longer so obvious because we are no longer directly affected by them. We no longer have to attend to the needs of our children, our laundry, or our cows; the concerns that call to us are those of the world.

Self-responsibility becomes global responsibility! How much need in the world can be addressed only by people who have enough time, money, and power? How much beauty and art can be created only by people who have enough leisure and peace? How much is there to repair, improve, complement, and renew in our world by men and women fortunate enough not to have to invest every waking minute in just staying alive?

We only have to develop a feeling for the Necessary, for the small, meaningful tasks all around us, waiting to be taken up, for the aesthetic potentials and ethical challenges we encounter every day. We must become aware of the hopes of the world, which are waiting for somebody to fulfill them. *It could be us* who in our spare hours fulfill hopes of the world.

This feeling for the Necessary has one presupposition: that we turn our attention away from ourselves. The insight gained from brain research in Vienna is related to the meaning crisis of our time: Self-transcendence spells success, whereas egocentricity leads to failure.

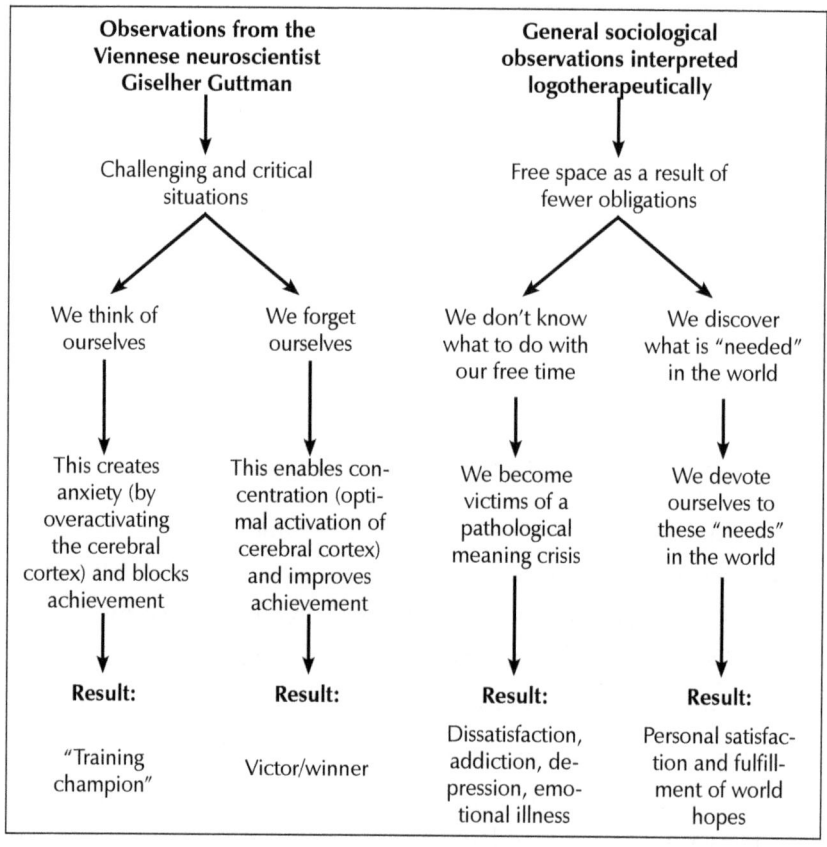

I refer again to the woman working only a few hours a week. She is probably bored during the remaining hours and wonders how to amuse herself. Amusement is all right, but the danger is that she will hop from party to party, from one fashion show to another, from one partner to the next, and in doing so feel progressively less entertained. The fear of missing something in life, of not getting enough out of life, will increasingly grip and spoil her joy in life. To express it in Guttmann's terms: Emotional factors will block her noëtic capabilities.

Therefore, it is better to focus on the people and the world around us and expand our awareness to include "need-turning" tasks, even if those needs do not directly affect us. Being aware of our global responsibility poses questions that are distinct from those of self-actualization. A nurse once said to me: "When I had to decide what kind of occupation to choose, I did not know what to choose at first. Then I wondered where I would be needed most, where there was a shortage of labor. All at once, I knew the answer." Not surprisingly, she is today one of the most sought-after nurses in a large Munich hospital.

The same point is made by the following dialogue reported by Liliane Giudice between a professor and a village pastor.[1] The professor saw a small girl who was badly disfigured playing in a meadow. He said to the pastor: "I'm sorry for the parents of this child." "Well," said the pastor, "her adoptive parents deserve admiration." The professor was surprised: "Adoptive parents? Who would adopt such a child?" The pastor replied: "The adoptive parents felt that precisely such a child should grow up with lots of love and care. That is why they welcomed her in their family." This demonstrates the recipe followed by those who pass the challenge; it is an illustration of global responsibility. Our town needs nurses? And I have to choose an occupation! This child needs loving parents? And we are in a position to adopt a child! Men and women who think in these terms feel what is necessary and fulfill hopes of the world.

THE FEELING FOR OTHERLINESS

The third area of sensitivity logotherapy wishes to encourage and develop is the feeling for Otherliness. In today's world we tend to live close together, which fosters aggression. And we live hectic and restless lives, which foments impatience. We have no time for each other and chafe against each other. Pick a family at random and observe the way its members talk with each other. You may be saddened. Pick a business organization at random and observe the way its members talk with each other. You may be shocked. Listen to the elite of our society who should be expected to converse in civilized, polite tones—you may be disappointed. Gentleness, compassion, understanding, and humor have all become rare qualities. Yet, to achieve a future worthy of human beings, little more is required than gentle, compassionate, understanding people, a twinkle in their eyes, telling us they can be trusted because they, in turn, trust others.

---

1 Giudice, L. (1981). *Oft ist es nur ein kleines Zeichen*. Heilbronn: Bugen Salzer.

Trust in others; what magic that word could work! Mountains of distrust would tumble, images of enemies would turn into mirages, and hate would burn itself out to become a curiosity. Trust in others would be a balm on every wound in the family, on every hurt inflicted in the business office, on every humiliation experienced during a lifetime. But this trust in others is a tender plant that thrives only in very special soil: It must be rooted in a feeling for the other person, a feeling for the Otherliness of the other person.

As a therapist who listens to people every day, I know from their tales what a large part those others play. But what is said about others is mostly bad. The others ought to be such and such, they should have done this, but they did that. The others are evil, they are the guilty ones; according to Jean-Paul Sartre, they represent hell on earth. No, in this soil our tender plant will not grow; in this hell, trust withers.

There is only one remedy. To let the others have their Otherliness and to accept it. For example, parents should keep in mind that their children differ from them, and that it is senseless to impose their own goals on the children. As children mature, they will also come to realize that their parents differ from them and there is no point in using their own perspective to judge their parents.

The evaluation of parents by their children is exploited in depth psychology rather uncritically for diagnostic purposes, but scientists have serious reservations about this. Of course, we all have something to forgive our parents for. But, then, we all have something to thank our parents for, too. And whether we remember the one or the other, whether we bring up one or the other in a depth-psychology session, depends on coincidences that can distort the entire evaluation.

In a partnership, it is equally important to allow the Otherliness of the partner to stand without being attacked, and to accept it with love. "Opposites attract," says the proverb. Yet opposites are also the seeds of conflict as soon as one partner wants to reshape the other's ideals according to his or her own. Khalil Gibran has wisely said that in a marriage, partners should swing in harmony like the strings of a lute but must never touch,

6. From Self-Actualization to Global Responsibility

none must pull the other over because, as the last distance between the two disappears, harmony is lost.

The Otherliness of the other person is not something that must just be tolerated: it is, instead, something to behold, something that, in fact, enriches the beholder. Our society would be poor, indeed, our culture monotonous, if we were all alike. But since we are all different, though equally valuable, we move in the center of a kaleidoscope of life that could not be more colorful and fantastic. We can enjoy this variety without manipulating or criticizing, we can refrain from persecuting the Otherliness and can extend our emotional antennae to probe and get to know it better. It would be rewarding, because what we know and understand we do not reject. If we are interested in a person we will not damn that person. The greater our empathy with others, the closer we are and the more related we feel, beyond all differences.

Paradoxically, the feeling for Otherliness is the only basis on which a feeling of having something in common can be built. As long as we see the Otherliness as alien, threatening, inappropriate, and undesirable, we will fight and reject it. We will not accept it; we will even prefer a division. But any division between the I and the You comes at the expense of the We. On the other hand, if we look at the Otherliness of others in love and respect, the alienation disappears and with it the division; the I and the very different You can be integrated in a common We.

For these reasons, logotherapy has been called an *agent of reconciliation*—something our generation and our general situation urgently needs. Logotherapy is a reconciler in three important areas: a) among academic disciplines, b) among various nations, and c) among various religions.

First, *logotherapy reconciles academic disciplines*. This is of considerable consequence in our era of specialization, in which professionals often know only their own special fields, and wear blinders to the rest. In my field, for example, there is mistrust between physicians and psychologists, between theologians and psychotherapists, between traditional doctors and holistic-health practitioners. But the world of tomorrow needs the cooperation of all disciplines; technology with ecology, biology with sociology, and so on. Logotherapy now unites different disciplines, especially those in the human sciences. Its tenets unite physicians and psychologists, ministers and educators, nurses and gerontologists. Logotherapy does not stress special techniques but principles of healing that help make life worth living, suffering tolerable, and human existence possible.

Second, *logotherapy is an agent of reconciliation in its potential to bring nations closer together*. Its basic principles focus on the specifically human—what differentiates us from animals and plants, and what is common in all humans regardless of nationality, class, stage of development, or mentality. The doctrine of the "specifically human" is more than a pious belief in all humans being equal. It is the doctrine of the actual equality of human nature, permitting us to find others in ourselves and ourselves in others, despite all otherliness.

Third, *logotherapy is an agent of reconciliation across religions*. It sees the spirit as the specifically human quality. This human spirit is not the spirit of our parents or forebears and certainly not of our animal ancestors. It has no material origin and therefore cannot decompose into matter. The spirit survives human graves. All religions have tried to express these mysteries in symbols. That's why logotherapy in its third function can reconcile the many religious communities. It subsumes ancient human wisdom in a scientific system which can be "translated" into any religious "language." It is a system that concentrates on something to which all can agree, regardless of what religious language they speak—as long as they raise their vision above material things. The feeling for Otherliness in a foreign religion is the only basis for the long-overdue discovery of what all religions have in common: the dialogue with divinity.

OUR PERSONAL CONTRIBUTION COUNTS

There exists a meaning of the moment, a demand of the situation for every human being everywhere and at all times. It is our responsibility to discover it and to respond to it. We are not only responsible for ourselves but, as a part of the world, we bear a global responsibility. This means we respond to the meaning of the moment—not merely in seeking self-actualization

6. From Self-Actualization to Global Responsibility

but in actualizing a future worthy of human beings. We choose to respond to the demand of the situation, not to benefit ourselves, but for a greater cause, although we cannot deny that we benefit in a humanly decent world in which good causes prevail.

To be ready and able to exercise this global responsibility calls for the expansion of three sensitivities: the feeling for the Sacred, the feeling for the Necessary, and the feeling for Otherliness. The feeling for the Sacred teaches us reverence for life, including one of our profoundest problems, the most effective protection against the destruction of the environment. The feeling for the Necessary teaches us self-limitation, which among other things is the most effective shield against uncontrolled population explosion, another challenging world problem. The feeling for Otherliness teaches us love for those close to us as well as for those far from us. Love is the best protective shield against war and violence, a still-unresolved world problem.

Let us begin, each day and in our small way, by shouldering our global responsibility. The demand of the situation is serious and *our personal contribution counts.*

What may we
expect of life?

The answer is silence.

What does life
expect of us?

The answer
lies on our tongue
and in our hand.

                          Elisabeth Lukas

CHAPTER 7

Correcting the Image

During the past few decades, many psychotherapeutic methods, techniques, and strategies have been developed, all aimed at restoring health in individuals with symptoms of psychological illness. Logotherapy is among these methods. However, it offers an addition that goes beyond analytical, heuristic, and behavioral techniques and will make it an essential approach for individuals in the 21st century.

Logotherapy introduces a *correction of the image*—the self-image of sick and healthy people, their image of the world, and, indirectly, even their image of God. By doing so, logotherapy not only draws attention to health, but also strengthens affirmative thinking, basic faith, and readiness for meaningful actions. This is accomplished through a philosophy and anthropology that views the human being in its existentiality: Logotherapy cures by letting people redefine themselves and others.

What this means in practice is easy to understand. We guide our lives by certain concepts of how we are allowed to act, how we ought to act, or how we must act, according to the values we attach to persons and things. If we see people in a negative light, we treat them with disdain or contempt. The same is true if we belittle ourselves—our decisions turn against ourselves. Broadly speaking, if we consider people as troublesome and evil, we become misanthropes.

In contrast, seeing people in their dignity and uniqueness helps us master even difficult human contacts. It also helps us accept ourselves and love others with their differences. This is essential in psychotherapy, but also in gerontology and in our relations with those who are sick and handicapped.

If we see people merely in a mechanistic or materialistic way, we see them, in effect, as a functioning machine that in sickness no longer functions properly and must be "fixed." This concentrates our thinking on "repair techniques" but does not strengthen our ability to love, to be patient, and to accept others when repair is not possible.

If we think there is little or nothing that can be done about a person—if any effort is considered "not worthwhile" because the person won't be able to become well again physically or psychologically—we give up. Such resignation becomes dangerous when economic, political, or societal considerations make the care of the sick person "cost ineffective."

Undoubtedly, logotherapy is the least mechanical or material-minded among all psychotherapeutic schools. Therefore, its image of the human being can be the model of a truly human anthropology.

Let us focus on problems that, according to all forecasts, are crucial in the 21st century, in the burgeoning field of gerontology. The increasing longevity of the population in technologically advanced countries poses a great challenge.

A significant number of older adults towards the end of life are chronically ill, in need of care, depressed, confused, and perhaps even a burden to their family. Someone has to attend to their needs. So both the caregivers and the cared for, the young and the old, are in distress.

Traditional psychotherapy has shown itself to be tentative about older adults. In contrast, logotherapy does not give up on them. Of course, logotherapy cannot compensate for losses, but that is not its focus. What is important to the logotherapist is the individual's self-image and the image of the world that is to be seen as meaningful up to the last moment. Here,

7. Correcting the Image

the logotherapist can reduce distress and therapeutically help caregivers as well as those who are receiving care. Frankl offers three specific "medicines": the presumption of a "what for," a last free area of choice, and the timeless purpose of caring for the departing.

THE PRESUMPTION OF A "WHAT FOR"

Any caring action presumes a Something for the sake of which the caring is done, or rather a Someone for whom it is done. Of course, it is done for the cared-for person. But it makes a big difference whether one sees this individual as a sick body with reduced brain capacity, or one looks, with something like X-ray eyes, through the frail organism to the intact human being in its deepest humanness. While nursing the organism, the presentation is from the worst side; with dirt, vulnerability, fragility. This does not make it easy to remain near and touch, especially when aesthetically disgusting factors bring on avoidance tendencies. One would prefer not to meet certain individuals who are aging. Nevertheless, they strongly need our presence; a touching hand or a word of sympathy is more important than any medicine. Intuitively, they feel from the reactions of others, regardless of whether they feel accepted as part of humankind.

Caregiving, such as cleaning, feeding, and dressing, is made easier if it is done for the sake of the spiritual human being, who exists beyond and above the sickness, who is infinitely more than a deteriorating organism, suffering from disability and weakness (without being identical to the disability and weakness). Such caregivers know the "what for" of the daily drudgery. They know for whom and for what they overcome their reluctance—a good feeling, in spite of many difficult hours!

THE LAST FREE AREA OF DECISION MAKING

Just as parents do not "create" their children, and physicians do not "create" the health of their patients, caregivers and family members do not "create" the well-being of those cared for. What caregivers can do is "throw the switches" toward desirable goals. This must be done in all modesty: They are allowed to pass something on into the hands of others—the hands of the cared for, hands that are greater than all the hands of the world.

A remnant of freedom remains in old age, in spite of the weaknesses of body and psyche, and despite the chaos of confused thoughts. The spiritual core of the human being can break through the walls of sickness and help shape patients' lives. If they do not want to feel well, no caregiver can please them. If they have turned away from their family, none of their members has a chance to reach them. This giving up of any desire to change, too, has to be respected in the caregiver's efforts to bring about changes.

Patients still retain a paper-thin area of decision-making, a remainder of being able to help shape their lives. If they are ready, even in their last phases, to listen and to respond to the call of meaning, they will find fulfillment, even when in a wheelchair or wrapped in covers in a bed; even when lacking the ability to see or hear well. Life is not so devoid of meaning that it can offer it only to the rich, beautiful, and strong.

It has been shown that caregivers and caring family members are less likely to suffer from burnout caused by disappointment and frustration if they do their service in the knowledge that the old and sick still have a last free area of decision making. Whether or not caregivers try is up to them; whether they succeed remains beyond their efforts. Those who are satisfied to have genuinely tried, aware of the human values of their patients, calmly do their work and reap the fruits of their work wherever those fruits evidence.

THE PURPOSE OF CARING FOR THE DEPARTING

We look not only for a what for, but also for a *why*. We want to know that, in the end, our efforts were not in vain. But the end of caregiving for the aging individual is death. The caregiver provides baths, dressings, massages, and a week later the individual is carried out in a coffin. Why the baths, dressings, and massages? A discouraging thought.

One may say that the patient during the last days still enjoyed a bit of a quality of life. Still, this argument smacks a bit of stale transitoriness. The feeling of well-being passes with breathtaking speed. Can it be that the entire goal of our strenuous effort of caregiving to the old is nothing but maintenance of a minimum quality of life?

7. Correcting the Image

To pay attention to the spiritual, noëtic dimension of people in their last phases of life is only a means, not an end. It is a means to allow individuals, in the noëtic dimension, to survey and to order their lives in order to bring them to a positive conclusion, to see what traces they have left in the world. If not distracted by pain, fears, and discomfort, the dying person can contemplate the meaning of the moment, which may be a last-minute reconciliation, a repentance, a love, a thanks rising in a heart preparing for departure. The dying are departing, preparing to return to their spiritual home and to take along what will be the eternal truth about themselves. Baths, dressings, massages, and other services only help them to "pack their luggage," to give them elbow room to forget their bedsores and wet diapers, to make peace and to find the one word or the one prayer that in the last analysis will have more weight than any lifelong failure.

Those who know they have accompanied others at the departure destined for a happy arrival, feel the "holiness" of their work and the reasons for doing it. They get a glimpse, while in their prime of life, of the light beyond the big, terrifying door.

>   Youth has many advantages
>   over old age:
>   It contains the seed
>   of its own future.
>
>   But one thing
>   youth never has:
>   the collected harvest
>   of a mature life.
>
>   — Elisabeth Lukas

CHAPTER 8

Overcoming the Tragic Triad: Suffering, Guilt, and Death

At a logotherapy conference, a participant handed me a Chinese saying: "We cannot do anything about the fact that the birds of worry and distress fly over our heads; we can, however, prevent them from building nests in our hearts." This saying is in keeping with logotherapeutic ideas, especially when it comes to the *tragic triad—suffering, guilt,* and *death*—which are part of the unalterable reality of our existence.

Even though the tragic triad represents a reality of our lives, saying that the birds of worry and distress must not build nests in our hearts means that we can apply the power of the human spirit to overcome the emotional distress which follows in the wake of suffering, guilt, and death.

SUFFERING

All suffering represents a loss. For example, a man suffering from serious illness has lost good health. A woman suffering because she cannot find a partner has lost hope for a fulfilling love relationship. A loss need not be irrevocable. A temporary loss of self-esteem, brought about by a long period of unemployment, can also result in acute emotional distress.

Logotherapy focuses less on the origin of suffering, and more on how to bear it. Frankl pointed out a direct connection between our ability to suffer and our basic attitude toward life. In the Logotest (which records attitudes toward life and investigates goals one has set oneself, whether one has reached them, and how to assess one's successes or failures) a young man wrote:

> I have reached almost all the goals I have set for myself, both privately and in school. School was a means to an end—to attain a position in life where I feel good. Life itself seems meaningless, but I am here whether I like it or not, so I want to make my time here as pleasant as possible. If anything were to upset my plans, I would regard it as a terrible blow.

These few sentences express his belief that life itself is meaningless, therefore it is to be made as pleasant as possible; if this fails, the consequences would be terrible! This results in a disastrous, though perfectly logical, chain of three links:

1. If life has no meaning, we transfer our attention to the direct pursuit of pleasure.
2. Pleasure, however, cannot be directly attained, but is the by-product of a meaningful activity or encounter; therefore we probably will not succeed in finding it.
3. If this is the case, a life without meaning and now also devoid of pleasure, becomes practically unbearable.

By joining the third link with the first, we realize that *our ability to bear suffering depends on the strength of our inner feeling of meaning fulfillment.* If we regard our lives as basically meaningful, we can put up with great suffering because life does not lose its meaning even if our pleasure has been diminished.

Individuals with an inner sense of meaning fulfillment are intuitively conscious of meaning. They sense it, take their bearings from it, and have something to search for. In peak moments they glimpse it, but it remains elusive. Those without this sense of meaning fulfillment do not even know what they are searching for and usually fail to find anything, Not having anything to search for is painful enough—but when, in addition, they experience a blow of fate, their capacity to carry burdens breaks down completely.

8. Overcoming the Tragic Triad

When we have lost our security because we doubt the meaningfulness of life, blows of fate are felt as dramatic voids in our existence.

Countless examples have shown that meaning can be perceived and fulfilled in spite of suffering, or even because of it. I remember a mother, Ms. A, who told me the story of her adopted daughter. After years of childless marriage, she became pregnant. Tragically, the child was stillborn. Ms. A lay in the hospital, weeping. In the next bed lay another woman, also weeping, although her newborn baby was perfectly healthy. She was a guest worker who had come to Germany to earn money. She became pregnant as a result of a moment of impulsiveness and could not return to her home with such a child. There the two women lay during those difficult hours, shattered to the very core of their being, yet connected by fate. Suddenly their individual suffering took on a common meaning: The guest worker gathered her courage and offered her baby to Ms. A, who accepted this little stranger with a heavy heart. This resulted in an adoption. When I saw the girl six years later, I saw a child who beamed at me through cheerful eyes, clearly happy and loved.

It looks like a happy ending but it came at considerable cost. The adopted girl was not a substitute for the stillborn baby, nor was parting with the little girl an ideal solution to the guest worker's problems. Nevertheless, there had been meaning in the way both women acted, a meaning borne out of the suffering they were forced to endure—a meaning which ultimately helped both to overcome their pain.

Another client lived in the country and suffered from a severe physical handicap which excluded him from many things in life. He said to me:

> You know, Dr. Lukas, even trees in dense forests that receive little light and warmth, and are thin and deformed, have their value. They provide wood for heating and offer us warmth and comfort in our homes. I can do the same, and that's all I want: to provide warmth even though fate has given me precious little of it.

Indeed, this man is held in high regard in his village because of his heart-warming manner.

These are immense achievements of the human spirit, examples of how loss can be overcome. They are borne out of the knowledge that everything contains meaning, one that can be extracted even in the face of utmost despair. I am not talking about putting up with suffering, repressing it, rationalizing it, or overcompensating for it; I am talking about an inner self-distancing that enables us to recognize meaningful structures that help us to transcend the situation. If we stand upright in the face of suffering we remain *above* suffering and become a towering example for others. We radiate a strength that spreads in the world around us and help others by our example; we invite others to imitate us.

There is, however, a kind of suffering that is self-made and contains no meaning. We all know individuals who put themselves into situations of suffering, whether for neurotic self-punishment, as a means of manipulating others, or simply out of resignation. Just about every form of addiction can be put into this category of self-inflicted suffering.

These persons do not have the problem of confronting fate or facing a loss; their problem is an inability to see and to actualize the positive possibilities life offers them. In these cases, inner meaning fulfillment plays an extended role: It does not enable them to bear suffering passively and it prevents them from actively inflicting suffering. There is a logical explanation for this. Meaning orientation enhances our ability to endure suffering because even a life darkened by suffering does not lose its meaning. But meaning orientation also inhibits our tendency to inflict suffering because a life not darkened by suffering gains meaning.

If we can overcome our self-hate, tame our manipulative impulses, or resist our tendency to become addicted, we have the chance of a richer, more fulfilled life. We can tackle plans that would have been out of the question, and we can open ourselves to experiences that were out of reach.

When we are confronted with suffering—our own, or of others—we need to remember that *life darkened by suffering does not lose meaning, and life not darkened by unnecessary suffering gains meaning.* If we bear this in mind, we will find it easier to abandon self-inflicted suffering and to pursue optimum attitudes toward the given circumstance.

GUILT

The complex subject of guilt comes under the heading of *overcoming failure*. Here we enter the realm of our personal past, for any current happening is still in the stage of development and cannot be called a failure before it has reached a conclusion. By failure, I mean *failure for which we are responsible*. Failures for which we are not responsible belong in the category of unavoidable suffering.

Regarding failures for which we are responsible, the gods are not very merciful: They rarely cover these failures with total oblivion; rather, they let a little tip show, which functions as a "guilty conscience." This does not necessarily mean that there is emotional damage. On the contrary, it might even lead to spiritual maturity. In logotherapy, guilt is looked upon as an opportunity to change, as an appeal to abandon old patterns and make new and better decisions. Therapists do not pass judgment but rather perform two functions.

First, together with their clients, they can explore whether or not the guilt feelings are justified. Together, they can ascertain whether the clients are responsible for what has happened or whether their failures can be attributed to factors beyond their control. We know that people often feel responsible for events that overwhelm them, even though they had little or no choice. Such events may justifiably cause anger or sorrow, but they must not be allowed to trigger feelings of failure. Should this be the case, therapeutic measures must be taken to counteract them.

The second function of the therapist is to help clients overcome failure when the sense of guilt is indeed justified. A therapist is not a Father confessor who can grant absolution. The so-called "psychological absolution" is too easy a way out: It requires virtually declaring the client incompetent, a helpless victim of powerful unconscious forces or conditioning processes that have formed the client's character.

There is another way of assisting without taking away the clients' spiritual freedom and dignity. In logophilosophy, we speak of an "optimism of the past," which regards the past as our "being" in its most genuine and concrete form. All things past are unchangeable; nothing can remove them. The future, in contrast, is rich in possibilities but devoid of actualities; it holds nothing final, every potentiality is only an opportunity which may or may not be taken. On the borderline between the nothingness of the future and the eternity of the past lies the present. We can never guarantee what will be actualized in the next moment. But what has been actualized a moment ago remains forever.

This means that the only sure thing that can really be called our own, the only reality that remains inseparably linked with our lives is what "has been." Take as an example an individual who has spent five years happily married. No power on earth can take those five years away, for they have been actualized, they have been "brought in as a successful harvest," as Frankl put it. Whether the person has 50 more years—or just one more day—of happily married life left is a question that remains unanswered. It is a question caught in a net of countless possibilities, none of which *is* yet an actuality and none of which, with the exception of one, will ever become one.

From this "optimism of the past" Frankl derived an "activism of the future." If eternity simply were to lie ahead of us, ready to unwind all by itself, we could just fold our arms and wait fatalistically for what lies ahead to happen. But because there is nothing ahead of us but unborn possibilities for whose selection we are responsible, we face the obligation to spot the most meaningful ideas, actions, and attitudes among the possibilities and to rescue them from the uncertainty of our future into the security of our past.

Guilt, therefore, can be seen as the result of a wrong choice, having actualized a possibility better left unchosen. But now it has become anchored in our past forever as an irreversible part of our life.

Seen this way, guilt is the converse of the optimism of the past; it is the "pessimism of the irrevocable." This is where the activism of the future comes in. Meaning can be found retroactively in all the good one did as a consequence of guilt, in every success learned borne out of failure, every positive opportunity seized because priority once had been given to a

8. Overcoming the Tragic Triad

negative one. Finding meaning retroactively can be seen as a correction of a previous wrong choice regardless of how irrevocable it was, because something meaningful cannot be entirely wrong.

Thus, we need not declare our clients incompetent and grant them psychological absolution. In fact, we *must not* declare them incompetent if we genuinely wish to help them overcome failure. Only those who are truly aware of their responsibility to choose among many possibilities—even possibilities that may lead from originally wrong choices to positive results—are in a position to resolve their guilt by revising their attitude toward it. In fact, we may find this insight reflected in the salvation myths of all great world religions. Only the relatively young science of psychology has disregarded it to date.

Just how unfortunate this disregard is, is shown by an experiment that has been carried out for many years on adolescents charged with crimes in my Munich counseling center. So-called "first timers," with the consent of the Juvenile Court, receive early release on condition that they participate in group therapy sessions. We are currently using the third approach for working with these delinquents and it would appear that we are now succeeding in keeping the rate of recidivism considerably lower than in previous years.

The first approach was based purely on social training. It failed because training assumes that participants bring sufficient motivation on their own to reach the training goal. Our clients did not have such motivation.

The second attempt sought to provide them with reasonable problem-solving strategies. Although they brought sufficient problems with them and were fairly motivated to work on solutions with the group leader, the problems discussed—mostly related to family and work—quickly became excuses for their faulty behavior. These excuses eliminated any possibility of finding meaning through subsequent correction of guilt.

In our third attempt, we applied logotherapeutic principles. We let guilt remain guilt, not as accusation or reproach, but as an opportunity to consider positive abilities, which each participant possessed regardless of environmental circumstances. We demonstrated to them that, just as they had been free to commit a wrong, so were they also free to do a meaningful deed. Soon after, a new attitude gradually worked its way through the mockery, scorn, disinterest, and demoralization. Occasionally, a participant used his or her freedom to do a meaningful deed. This encouraged the others, and gradually the change in attitude lead to a change in behavior. Granted, the path is rocky, and there are setbacks, but this path clearly leads to overcoming failure.

DEATH

Logotherapy has given much attention to death. Here the issue is *overcoming transitoriness*. We are dealing with the question of how to handle our knowledge that we are mortal. No other living creature is required to carry this burden. Logotherapy once again relies on its optimism of the past and points out that nothing can take away the valuable things we have done and which are irretrievably anchored in our past. Every task we have fulfilled, every happy experience, every suffering courageously borne, every guilt redeemed in a mature manner—all these things have become part of the eternity of the past, the essence of our being, the quality of our life, our identity. None of this can be taken away from us, even long after we have returned to dust.

When we discuss such ideas with clients, they often question whether the events of their lifetime have not become irrelevant by the time nobody knows anything about them any longer. "What difference does it make," they ask, "whether I have lived a good life or whether I suffered courageously when nobody remembers me after my death?" Yes, everything is forgotten; nothing earthly can be remembered forever. But what is past still remains as it was; the fact that it is no longer remembered cannot wipe it out.

Frankl wrote: "Thinking of something cannot make it happen; by the same token, no longer thinking of something cannot destroy it." It remains. Whether the level of its quality makes any difference is a question that we can only answer through faith. But our deep longing for salvation and our existentially rooted search for meaning indicates that *what* has remained of each of us in our past *does* matter.

8. Overcoming the Tragic Triad

A CASE HISTORY

I would like to conclude these philosophical considerations with a case history that illustrates the "tragic triad." A married couple sought my advice in a rather delicate matter. Ms. D, who wore mourning clothes, told me that a few days ago her aging mother had died after a long sickness. The problem was not the loss of the mother, which had been expected, but whether the father of Ms. D should be told of his wife's death. When I asked how it was possible that he did not know about it, I received the following explanation:

The parents had been married for many decades and had truly loved each other. When Ms. D's mother became sick, the father took care of her and refused any help from others. Taking care of his wife became the content of his life, his personal task. But three weeks earlier he suffered a heart attack and had to be hospitalized. At present, he remained in critical condition in intensive care. It was not certain how much he knew about what was going on, as he was mostly unconscious, but occasionally he seemed to indicate that he was bothered by something. He often played with his wedding ring; Ms. D suspected that he was worried about being sick when his wife needed him.

The doctors advised not to tell the critically ill man the bad news because they feared the shock would kill him, and they wished to spare the dying man that last pain.

The arguments of the physicians were plausible but let's consider the old man's situation from the point of view of the "tragic triad" and how he might overcome it. His future held little hope. He was bound to die of heart failure, and if a brief respite should be granted to him, he would return to an empty apartment and mourn his wife.

In contrast, the realities of his past were that he had lived a full life, faithfully worked in his job, fought through the bad years, enjoyed the good ones, and devoted his last years to his wife. He had actualized a rich human existence on which he could look back with satisfaction and pride Only one bitter pill was left, one task had not been completed: The care of his wife, in his eyes, was not finished. Here he might feel failure—the worry about the beloved partner may rob the dying man of inner peace, and not let him die peacefully. Ms. D sensed it, she knew her father well enough to guess what was happening in his mind.

I advised her, contrary to the recommendations of the physicians, to let the father gently know that his wife had preceded him and that he didn't need to worry about having left her behind. This, we hoped, would help him see that he had also fulfilled his last task, and he would be able to close his eyes in peace.

I must admit that I felt doubts when I let the couple go from the counseling session. We can never be entirely sure if the meaning we have read into a situation objectively was "meant" by the situation or if we subjectively have decided to consider it meaningful.

In this case, I received positive feedback. Mr. D let me know that his father-in-law had received the news of his wife's death calmly. He had nodded his head several times and whispered: "That's good; now I'll join her."

After that, he lived longer than the physicians expected. He slept most of the time with a relaxed expression on his face. When he died, the fingers of his right hand clasped his wedding ring.

8. Overcoming the Tragic Triad

Two gates:
Through one we are pushed;
through the other we may pass.
Are these gates in contradiction?
Perhaps.
But they are connected
through our steps.

One is called Fate,
the other, Freedom.

One shows us the direction
we must go; the other allows us
to choose the path we take.
While walking, we may choose,
but while we choose we must
keep on walking.

Two gates,
two worlds,
and people on their thresholds—
wavering between fate and freedom?
Not quite.

Because being pushed
through the gate of fate,
leaves fate behind us,
but being allowed to enter
through the gate of decision,
we face our freedom.

Thus, we walk upright,
fate in back,
toward freedom.

Elisabeth Lukas

CHAPTER 9

"Key words" as a Guarantee Against the Imposition of Values by the Therapist

As a therapeutic approach that provides meaning and value-oriented support in all aspects of life, the application of logotherapy is applied not only to anxiety syndromes, affective disturbances, addictions, sexual aberrations, and personality and behavior disturbances; it can also support young people in their search for themselves and in their efforts to reach maturity. It can help the elderly to look back on their lives to prepare for departure. It can guide lovers and family members through conflicts, and help working people as well as the unemployed to cope with the demands placed on them, whether too great or too little. It can even raise up those who are bent under their cares and resentments, and lead people who have lost their spiritual home back to their ideal roots.

Logotherapy can do all of this; yet its only medium is language. If we disregard its content for the moment, it is a therapeutic–pedagogical–philosophical–pastoral dialogue form. The critical examination of patients' statements does not mean that the therapist gives a lecture. Logotherapy takes the form of a dialogue, an exchange of ideas that entwines itself around the patient's statements in a joint effort to reach a consensual understanding of a piece of truth. It aims at helping individuals to better understand the meaning opportunities that await them in the world. For this purpose, the therapist introduces ideas, helps to think through possible consequences, and stimulates the patient spiritually.

The danger exists, however, that the therapist could make judgments on what is right and wrong in patients' lives and impose the therapist's own value standards on them. Frankl often stated that the external imposition of values on patients would totally contradict his intentions.

LOOKING FOR CUES

If we assume that conscience is the meaning organ of the human being, then it is comparable to a prompter, giving us cues to tell us in which directions we should take actions in order to seize the opportunities for the meanings demanded from us. Each situation demands that we apply a certain value standard. But the values against which this standard is calibrated are anchored in such a deep layer of our being that we can do nothing but follow them unless we wish to risk being untrue to ourselves.

In light of these considerations, the optimal success of therapy would mean that the participants reach the stage where they could do nothing (or wish nothing) except to follow conscience, whose standards are based on their innermost value standards. Whenever we work with people, especially with persons who are suffering, it is important to listen for a cue, a *key word* that will unlock the chamber where the hidden cares are kept. When the key word opens the door, then values shine through, and the voice of conscience whispers more audibly. This allows the therapist to adapt arguments that prompt patients to correct their behavior and attitudes in line with their own convictions. The logotherapist has to listen for signals from the deepest (or "highest") plane of the client, to listen to what the noëtic person is saying.

THE PROBLEM OF AMBIVALENCE

Ambivalence means liking *and* disliking contrary possibilities. Patients do not formulate a clear "yes" or "no" in their hearts. The resulting long-term inner state can be extremely unpleasant, since all activities undertaken in

9. "Key Words" as a Guarantee Against the Imposition of Values

this connection are overshadowed by a lack of a clear sense of purpose; in these situations, energy is blocked.

For example, an acquaintance offers Marie, a young woman in Sicily, a job in a pizzeria in Munich. She is a widow with a small child, and is unemployed. If she does not accept the job, she will pass up the opportunity to earn an adequate income and offer her child better opportunities. If she goes to Munich, she will have to leave the child with relatives and live on her own in a foreign city, where she does not speak the language. Both alternatives seem bleak. Finally, she heeds the urgings of her acquaintance and moves to Munich, where she sits and cries all day. If she had decided to stay in Sicily, she would have reproached herself for turning down a good source of income. Unhappiness is inevitable in either case.

How is therapeutic help possible? It is not permissible for the therapist to make value judgments that point in one direction or the other—at least not until the therapist has decoded which of the alternatives barely "tips the scales" in favor of meaning for the patient. Who tells the therapist? The patients themselves.

I asked Maria: "What actually caused you to choose the pizzeria in Munich?"

Maria replied: "In Sicily, there is severe unemployment. I would like to have enough money so my son can receive the best possible education to find good work later."

I then asked what she could do for her son if she were to return to Sicily. She replied, "Not much. Apart from my presence, I couldn't offer him much."

"But isn't your presence something very precious for the child, too?"

She: "Yes, of course, but it can be replaced, because my son is very close to his grandparents, aunts, and cousins."

From this dialogue we can gather that there was a nuance that tipped the scale in favor of Munich. Maria saw a good education for her son as more valuable than her motherly presence, which she even called "replaceable."

After careful listening to Maria, I reinforced this tiny hint of the greater value of one alternative so she could make a more unequivocal affirmation of her decision.

I surmised: "So you believe that your son will suffer little and profit greatly in the long term through your absence because you are earning money. And you think that this combination of suffering little and profiting greatly can only be reached through your great suffering here in Munich?"

Maria reflected and agreed, to which I said, "Why aren't you proud of yourself then instead of crying?" I challenged her. "Why don't you say to yourself every day in the pizzeria when you are peeling potatoes and vegetables; 'I'm doing this for you, my son!' Later, when you are learning vocabulary lists in your rented room, why don't you say again, 'I'm doing this for you!' Later still, when you pick up your salary from the bank, say, 'This is for your future, my son. Earned through your mother's efforts….'"

Almost any mother would breathe more easily on hearing such words. Maria saw that she was on the right path. Here, "right" referred to her own convictions and not to mine. Ambivalence can be resolved only through intensive discernment of every tiny nuance, every small hint of "moreness" that speaks in favor of one alternative over the other in terms of values. Did the child's future opportunities outweigh the mother's present fears? Yes, they did—the clear "yes" had been regained by Maria herself.

THE PROBLEM OF NONACCEPTANCE

Some people react to a challenge of fate with a rebellion that sooner or later hardens into an attitude of stubborn refusal. Those who are mired in a state of stubborn protest can be moved to adopt an attitude of flexible acceptance only if they abandon their perspective of personal deprivation and turn to a viewpoint that is receptive of values. In such cases, the therapist must intensify the perception of those who constantly protest and refuse to accept something—but the therapist also has to make sure that no externally imposed values are pushed into the field of perception. This again demands that we cautiously grope our way in the direction of the signals sent out by the patients.

9. "Key Words" as a Guarantee Against the Imposition of Values

An example: Carla was separated from her parents as a child during the chaotic period after the war. She lived in a convent children's home until her mother was found. Her father had been killed in the war. At the age of 30, Carla attempted to join a religious order but was not accepted. Her wish was dismissed as a passing whim or a spiteful reaction following an unhappy love affair. Carla was deeply insulted by this rejection and could not get over it. She felt that the religious order had failed to recognize her religious motivation, and had chased her away like a stray dog. She was frozen in silent protest.

During our conversations, I took up this lack of recognition of her motivation. "What would you honestly say you were looking for in the convent?" I asked.

"Security," she answered simply.

"You are bitter because you did not get what you were looking for?" I persisted.

"Does that surprise you?" she retorted.

"Well," I answered, "actually you got security, but years earlier, as a child. Back then, when you were suddenly alone in the world, a convent gave you shelter. Who knows what would have become of you? The convent also searched for your mother. So you would be within your rights to say: 'What I was looking for in the convent at the age of 30 was granted to me a child. The fact that I was once in a convent, and secure, can never be taken away, not even by a Mother Superior.'"

Carla laughed. "That is a liberating thought!" she called out, "Of course one could also look at it that way!" And she added, "Perhaps being sheltered in a convent twice would have been too much of a good thing, what do you think?"

I had no trouble agreeing with her.

The following example is more tragic: Michael was in a coma for five days after a motorcycle accident. Thereafter, he was seriously disabled; many physical movements were no longer possible. The work to regain movement cost him unimaginable efforts for microscopic progress. He was desperate. What is more, he had an irrational grudge against his parents who had bought him the motorcycle. It had been second-hand, and Michael was obsessed with the notion that the brakes would have worked better on a new motorcycle, if only his parents had been less interested in saving money. This was his way of compensating for his own share of the blame; according to the police report, Michael had been speeding on a bad road.

It was understandable that Michael did not wish to accept his situation. On the other hand, it would remain unendurable if he did not achieve final acceptance and, in fact, he harbored a desire to die. All of his hopes were gone. For many hours, I merely listened to his complaints. I was waiting for something, but I did not know what.

One afternoon it came. It was a memory of a plan in the past to attend a climbing course. Shortly before his accident, he had obtained brochures from several schools in the Alps that offered such courses. I leafed through them with him. Sitting in his wheelchair, he could hardly hold them steady. The photographs of mountain climbers daringly scaling treacherous cliff faces set his cheeks aglow. "Fantastic!" he murmured to himself, "Awesome!"

That was my cue. "Oh yes," I agreed. "Mountain climbers master great challenges. But that is nothing compared to what you are up against. The rock that you are climbing step by step in physical therapy is higher than the highest mountain in the world. No one has reached that peak before you, because no one has been in exactly the same situation. The steep walls before you seem insurmountable. No steps, no handholds in sight. But have the courage to climb anyway! You wanted to learn to climb—now you have a chance as never before to master a great climbing challenge! Prove to yourself that you won't surrender. Fight your desire to quit, carry the flag to the top and plant it on the peak of your triumph over weakness and infirmity."

The young man closed the brochure in his hand and pressed it to his chest. "That's a way I could imagine giving myself another chance," he whispered to himself, "but will I make it?" I got up and bent over to him. "You are climbing with an invisible rope which holds you up, I'm sure of that." With these words I left him to his inner images.

9. "Key Words" as a Guarantee Against the Imposition of Values

Since then, Michael has been on the road to improvement. He no longer mentions the wish to die and has come to terms with his parents. He manages his daily exercises with relentless energy. And he always keeps a brochure from a climbing school in his room. He has become one of the most admirable "climbers" I know,

In both of these cases, people moved forward from frozen attitudes of protest to more flexible postures of acceptance. It was not the power of persuasion that made this possible. I did not impose the value judgment on Carla to see the convent as a place where security can be found, or the enthusiasm for mountain climbing as an act of Michael proving himself. I read these from their own statements and used them to heal spiritual wounds. I injected them with that which, in logotherapeutic terms, was already in them.

THE PROBLEM OF INDIFFERENCE

Among the least promising therapeutic undertakings is working with people who are walled in by indifference. Whatever the approach taken, they do not respond spiritually because a hard shell of ignorance or even brutality surrounds the soft core of their inner being. They established this shell to protect them in earlier phases of their lives, and it remains with them.

But how can they get rid of it? There seems to be hardly any effective remedy. Those who ignore their fellow human beings, lose their sense of awe, or break all rules of decency increasingly exclude themselves from human society and then need an even thicker shell. Soon they don't have contact with their inner selves, let alone with others. The gentle stirrings of the spirit are left to waste away in a vacuum of values.

If we are fortunate, however, the shell has cracks in which a deep longing for a meaningful existence gathers. By driving a wedge in at these places, we can occasionally chip away a piece of the shell and create space for new sensitivity to develop.

Julia, an individual with morbid obesity, complained incessantly. Her crisis had been triggered by a company excursion during which she had quarreled with her supervisor. Because her colleagues had taken his side, she had lost her temper and threatened to file suit for slander. As a consequence, she was dismissed after ten years of loyal employment, or so she claimed.

I asked her to describe the excursion in detail. The program had been planned by the supervisor: a bus trip, a walk up to a recently renovated castle on a hill, lunch at the castle, chamber music in the concert hall of the castle, a walk down the hill to the bus for the return journey. A pleasant program. "Very pleasant!" said the patient scornfully. "We had to trudge all the way up the stupid hill. How can anyone think up such a stupid trip? The route was stupid, the supervisor was stupid."

"Did everyone on the trip think that?"

"No," she screamed in my face. "The others hopped from stone to stone like young deer while the sweat was pouring into my eyes and my blouse was clinging to me. I could hardly get my breath. It was pure torture!"

"For you!" I said emphatically.

"Yes, for me "

"For you, and not for the others." I repeated.

Julia was silent tor the first time. "Could it be your obesity that caused your problems?"

"And what if it did" she grumbled in a more moderate tone. "I'm just too stupid to control my eating. I've tried all kinds of ways and have never stuck with it. I just can't. "

The cat was out of the bag. "You're angry about your past inability to lose weight," I said, summing up the situation, "and that makes you malicious. The route is stupid. The supervisor who planned it is stupid. You yourself are stupid in your eyes. And getting fired is the most stupid thing of all. Anger makes you ignorant. You ignored the fresh forest air, the beauty of the castle, the concert, and the friendly organizers, You were too busy fending off your real problem." I got out paper and a pencil. "Now correct what is not right in your soul and in your thoughts. Write down: 'The route to the castle was inspiring. My supervisor chose it with wise foresight. I myself am a nice woman with all kinds of talents. The only bothersome thing is

9. "Key Words" as a Guarantee Against the Imposition of Values

my obesity. However, I have a new opportunity to fight it. My dismissal is a chance to change my eating habits. I will use the time I now have on my hands to go on a diet. After this I will look for a new job and nothing in my life is stupid anymore.'"

"You want me to write that?" she asked in astonishment.

But she did as I told her and took the page home.

The result?—Unfortunately, not a slim person; but nevertheless something positive came of it. When she began her next job she wrote her former supervisor a letter of apology and sent me a copy. In it she wrote, "You planned a wonderful excursion with a completely suitable route. It was my fault that I couldn't jump like a young deer. Forgive me." Now, in a certain sense, the patient did manage to jump in the end, namely over her own shadow and over her emotional defenses.

It is hard to help people who ignore and trample on all that is valuable in their surroundings. If it is at all possible, then it is so only through persistent questioning of their justifications for demolishing their will to meaning.

A drop of blood
caused by a small wound
is hardly felt.

A drop of a tear
caused by a small pain
is hardly noticed.

A drop of bitterness
in a glass of sweet wine
is hardly tasted.

A right word
spoken at the right moment
can say everything.

Elisabeth Lukas

CHAPTER 10

A Person's Admission Into Self-Responsibility: Reducing the Relapse Rate in Psychotherapy

Viktor Frankl's logotherapy is not merely one among many forms of psychotherapy, as if it were just one individual link in a very long chain of psychological theories; it is also a *starting gate for the development of human maturity*. It has the anthropological foundations with which to raise the level of maturity of a person. That distinguishes it from other psychotherapeutic formulations, which only have the tools to lead a person to a stage of emotional stability. In fact, the directional goal of logotherapy goes beyond the usual wish to cure. The deepest concern of logotherapy is not only to cure, but to "cure once and for all." This is because every increase in spiritual maturity logically contains within itself the promise of making further therapy unnecessary, because the individual's newly acquired maturity enables the person to deal meaningfully with future crises.

Logotherapy is the—perhaps the only—psychological concept that can counter the increase of psychological disturbances in the population, and of the emergence of more and different forms of therapy—which may each be in a reciprocal relationship. Logotherapy ends the problematic necessity of "more and more" psychotherapy and dramatically reduces the relapse rate, which amounts to a revolution. In order to understand the importance of this statement, it is important to remember that the practice of psychology currently depends *mainly* on "long term patients," from those who come for counseling more or less regularly. And even when their treatment has long since been completed, they reappear years later looking for further advice and help.

This can be explained by the fact, that whatever kind of help is given, a *dependency* on this help also arises. Individuals in treatment ultimately believe that they could most easily solve their problems if they have help in solving them. As well, there is a risky but unavoidable *hyperreflection*[1] that results from intense focus during therapy about past and present life crises and which anchors the person in an immature egocentricity. Even "solved" problems are and remain at least "past" problems and always leave behind the bitter aftertaste of the fear they could re-emerge.

Along with such inner dispositions that are present in individuals, predisposing them for a relapse, external factors must be considered. These factors are like handcuffs for emotionally unstable persons and can easily make them fall again. An accident, a blow of fate, a serious loss— or simply the fact of becoming older and weaker—can throw a neurotic or depressive person back into neurosis and depression, even when undergoing expensive treatment for years. What is tragic in that is both: The patients are happy to be able in a situation of need to return to the same counselors who have perhaps already helped them many times; and the therapists in general have nothing against keeping their patients, because for them a good income is secured.

However, all this does not happen in the interest of a spiritually mature society, for it keeps sickness in a state of flux rather than a state of health. A healthy society is composed of self-responsible individuals, who decide the sphere of interest in their lives and who accept the consequences of their conduct. If the percentage of immature, helpless, and emotionally ill people in a society substantially increases, then the entire society runs into danger, and indeed into greater danger than if it were threatened by an enemy from outside. What can help is not an army of psychotherapists

---

1 A logotherapeutic term, meaning excessive attention. First defined by Viktor E. Frankl (1947). *Die Psychotherapie in der Praxis.* Vienna: Franz Deuticke.

10. Admssion Into Self-Responsibility: Reducing the Relapse Rate

or a flood of psychological techniques, but simply initiating a process of spiritual maturation, for which logotherapy is uniquely suited.

The following *four-stage program*, which I would like to introduce as a way into self-responsibility, implies one such possibility of curing patients "once and for all" and thus of crucially reducing the percentage of emotionally ill people in the society.

The *first stage* of my program is well known. Briefly, it is the level of *symptom reduction and problem solving*, which of course has priority above all else; the acute misery of the individual must be alleviated. In my practice, I work at this level in one-on-one sessions. People must be able to trust and to show themselves and also to expose their most intimate problems or desires, those not intended for any other person. In my opinion, it is not useful to force individuals at this stage to discuss their difficulties within a group; individuals are still tightly bound up with their own problems and would all too easily relate the problems of the other group members to themselves in a negative way. The benefit from hearing that other people also have their problems is small, and the knowledge of how much worry and sorrow there is all around us only promotes a pessimistic attitude which does not serve the process of cure.

As well, patients at the first stage, who are still struggling with their weakness and troubles, have much too little detachment from themselves and their situation to profit from group discussions. They may become insecure when they hear what the group says and experience their own "revelations" sometimes as degrading, something which should never happen in psychotherapy. The dignity of the person must remain unimpugned.

In the individual sessions, all *specifically logotherapeutic methods* that fit the symptoms can be applied. Here, paradoxical intention can be employed with various forms of anxiety and obsessions, dereflection can be applied to autonomic and psychosomatic disturbances, and attitude modulation to depressive and negativistic tendencies.[1] At this stage, it is critical to create

---

[1] Logotherapeutic methods are detailed in Frankl, V. E., (1986). *The doctor and the soul* (2nd ed.). New York: Vintage Books/Random House and Lukas, E. (2019). *Meaningful living: Introduction to logotherapy theory and practice*. Charlottesville: Purpose Research.

as much inner detachment as possible between the spiritually intact areas of patients and their emotional overreactions and false reactions; only out of such detachment can patients put up resistance even under the most unfavorable conditions. We must encourage healthy resistance in every way, if we are to free individuals from the grasp of illness and return them to a normal, healthy life.

In addition, other techniques can be combined with logotherapy at this first stage; for example, logotherapy can be used with behavior therapy, suggestion methods, and relaxation techniques, as well as with the purposeful use of psychopharmaceuticals. This stage primarily involves symptom reduction, and we do not at all need to be ashamed of that. It is often much more difficult to actually bring a symptom to extinction, than to design bold hypotheses about its origin and development, irrespective of the fact that the patient is suffering from the symptom the same as before.

The first stage is usually concluded with partial success, insofar as those problems which were changeable have been reduced or solved, while the rest of the problems remain which are unchangeable at the time. What also remains is an unavoidable hyperreflection about the suffering experienced as a result of other problems. This is a hyperreflection that would—were patients at this stage released as cured—(mis)lead them into again observing their deepest feelings and particular circumstances in the most exact way out of fear that they would not be able to cope with life. But *fear produces what is feared*. Logotherapy has taught us that often enough, and therefore we know that it is dangerous to release patients with ongoing hyperreflection out into life. Even if they feel good and seem to be free of symptoms, we should never forget that a cure at this stage is in every case a potential relapse. That is also the reason why I turned to building a *second therapeutic stage: general dereflection*.

While logotherapy in the first stage offered orientation assistance through its very specific tactics and theory of neurosis, it now helps at this second step through its theory of the human being. All who are familiar with logotherapy know that Viktor Frankl sketches human beings as "beings in search of meaning," equipped with the capacity for self-transcendence, by means of which it is possible for them to comprehend and to shape the world around them. But every unhealthy egocentricity, which is necessarily bound up with the phenomenon of hyperreflection, weakens self-transcendence and consequently clouds the view of the external world, which can almost no longer be comprehended and can already no longer be shaped.

It is therefore important to lift up the persisting hyperreflection in the form of a general dereflection, to loosen the egocentricity and to strengthen the self-transcendence, so that the full meaningfulness of life can once again be perceived. Then and only then is a person able to "reach with both hands" into this perceived meaningfulness and to find new personal goals and ideals within it.

Such a general dereflection should not be confused with the method of specific dereflection for overcoming sleep or sexual disturbances at the first step. The general dereflection of the second stage is not in any way used for symptom reduction, but rather for bringing about a disinterest in all symptoms. This is brought about by helping individuals to consciously look away from present and past problems and instead to turn to the positive and creative areas of their lives. I use general dereflection in a group to take advantage of the high probability of members supporting each other in their efforts to direct their attention to what is positive. We begin the group (made up only of persons who have mostly completed the first stage) with a certain stipulation, namely the agreement that participants are allowed to talk about whatever they want, but not about something which is negative for themselves. This is a matter of intentionally ignoring problems in order to hinder the unproductive mulling over problems and to counteract the hyperreflection.[1]

That is not at all a "repression" of problems; there is always the offer of a one-on-one session with the therapist for clarifying any crisis situation which comes up. Besides, the participants of the dereflection group are already past problem clarification, at least as far as that is possible. Now they have the

---

1 A detailed description of an early dereflection group can be found in Chapter 6, pp. 87-99 of Lukas, E. (2015). *Meaning in Suffering*. Charlottesville: Purpose Research. —Ed.

task of newly building their future lives in view of their former illness and in view of fateful aspects that may be lasting. The goal of the dereflection group is rather to follow the *logotherapeutic imperative*, which means that the psychotherapist only has to make what is unconscious conscious, in order to finally let it become unconscious again. Thus the therapist always has to reestablish the obviousness of unconscious processes. Everything that had to be brought into consciousness for the purpose of therapy at the first stage, and all the difficulties which caused the patient so much trouble earlier, should now gradually become unimportant, forgotten or at least incidental, because of the compensating power of the positive, which makes it relative.

Most often, I have found that as soon as group participants become familiar with our stipulations, they are seriously and spontaneously committed to eliminating the negative thoughts from the center of their conversations. Yet they just sit there, quiet and still, because something which is not negative does not spontaneously arise in their thoughts at this point. From their staring, we can see the enormous hyperreflection in which they are trapped, and it certainly requires therapeutic skill to overcome this inertia.

In my practice, I use various means to this end; for example, reading aloud a contemplative poem, reflection on a beautiful bouquet of flowers, or listening to an impressive piece of music, after which conversations with a positive focus flow more easily. There are also supportive exercises for improving our perception of values, for example, word association exercises, in which the participants close their eyes a few minutes and associate positive experiences or encounters from their lives to a given word, in order to speak about it afterwards.

After four or five group sessions, the inertia is overcome and the patients bring increasingly positive contributions into the group; they are learning in their everyday lives to pay more attention to what is positive. They keep diaries of nice experiences, in which they make notes of the small high points of their lives, or at night before they go to sleep they recapitulate what was pleasant during the day in spite of everything. Because talking about something negative is allowed as long as the participant has succeeded in transforming this negative into something positive, they offer encouraging models for each other in the art of coping with life. Sometimes they develop admirably courageous attitudes, which the therapist could not better express.

In case group members ignore the stipulation and fall back into complaining or feeling sorry for themselves, discussion of the topic is ended and they are given a "special assignment," which must be completed by the next session. Usually this means that they should find out how they could consider their own topic from a more optimistic perspective. Sometimes true wonders happen here, insofar as even persistent pessimists suddenly recognize the good sides of life, and those who were constantly dissatisfied now exercise forgiving in a most generous way.

However, when the dereflection group proceeds well, the stipulation is seldom ignored; the participants themselves soon strictly adhere to the basic agreement and support each other in their struggle to see what is valuable. For example, one member may tell other participants where their strengths lie and motivate them to further develop these strengths and to make them useful in other parts of their lives. In this way, the hyperreflection of one's own weakness automatically passes into the background and fades.

By the end of the dereflection group no one identifies with the label of "emotionally ill" any more. The group members no longer see a mountain full of problems in front of themselves. Quite the opposite; each person has rather the liberating feeling of standing high up on a mountain peak and viewing all the paths down below, which could lead to positive goals. But patients at this second stage do not give themselves up to illusions. They know that there will be obstacles in their paths and that some paths may turn out to be dead ends. But they also know that they have certain healthy forces in them which enable them to climb over obstacles and that there are directional signs in the environment which show the way out of the dead-end streets.

If they have learned at the first stage to cope with life to a certain extent, then they learned at the second stage to comprehend life as positive and meaningful. If pressed for time, it can be justified to release a participant as "cured" at this second stage back into life. But if we want to reduce the danger of relapse to an absolute minimum, then we should not do without the *third stage*, which has a future-oriented function: it serves exclusively for *prophylaxis*.

Earlier it was noted that there were, above all, two types of dangers for relapses. The first involves unfavorable inner dispositions in those who are to be released, and the other relates to the external causal factors that could fatefully overwhelm them and throw them back into their illness. Inner dispositions such as hyperreflection, anticipatory fears, or pessimistic basic attitudes largely can be weakened in the dereflection group. But no therapist can keep the danger of external blows of fate away from patients. There will be occupational complications, family conflicts, economic limitations, personal losses, even illness and the threat of death in the life of every patient. How will individuals react? Will they survive the storms of life unscathed or will they again fall prey to despair, from which the therapist has just torn them away with the greatest of difficulty? In order to prevent the latter, I invite the cured patients to participate at the third stage in a *logotherapeutic meditation group*, which has a different intention than the dereflection group.

While logotherapy at the first stage offers us special methods and therapeutic techniques, and at the second supports us with its positive theory of the human being, it now places at our disposal its *philosophical principles*. These are principles which strengthen our backbone just in that moment when fate becomes a frontal attack. We present-day specialists know logotherapy as an efficient therapy which has proven itself in our daily practice. But we should not forget that its philosophical foundation has also been proven somewhere else, namely in the chaos of a concentration camp during the Second World War. Thus from the cradle on, logotherapy has a very special power to encounter fate in an optimal manner. If there is a psychotherapy which is able to offer consolation, it is logotherapy. And if there is a psychotherapy which can succeed in immunizing its patients prophylactically against falling into despair with the blows of fate, then it is also logotherapy.

10. Admssion Into Self-Responsibility: Reducing the Relapse Rate

This special power of logotherapy is used at the third stage to awaken certain attitudes by means of meditations using vivid symbols and imagery. These attitudes should make it possible for them to cope later on with any situation of life. In every group session, the therapist introduces an image or a symbol from the treasury of logotherapeutic concepts. A group discussion ensues during which criticism may be expressed, but only constructive criticism. In general, however, I have never met with strong rejection. On the contrary, the lively and exciting discussions and the intensive reflections of the participants on the symbols and coping aids offered prove their deep commitment.

One of the first and most suitable images to be discussed by the meditation group is the *three-dimensionality of human existence* and the superiority of the defiant power of the human spirit[1] in relation to the pressure of emotional needs. The symbol of an airplane that is able to move on the ground like an automobile but which becomes fully an airplane only when it lifts itself into the air, beautifully illustrates that human beings are only fully and truthfully human, when they rise to the heights of the spiritual dimension.

We can add here the logotherapeutic principle that happiness or pleasure cannot be directly pursued, but rather ensue as a side effect, when a spiritual goal is the focus of intention. In discussing this phenomenon, we can offer many examples from the area of sexuality and love, the area of occupational success and power, or from the area of self-actualization. The symbol of the eye which is sick when it sees itself, as in cataracts, and which is healthy when it sees everything but itself, fits in perfectly.

After these exercises we can gradually proceed in the meditation group to a discussion of the logotherapeutic *triad of values* and encourage participants to produce their own ideas for creative values, experiential values, and attitudinal values. Here the special position of the attitudinal values soon crystallizes, namely their heroism and their enormous positive radiance. Whoever actualizes attitudinal values in the logotherapeutic sense is

---

1 Refers to the noëtic freedom to take a stand toward all conditions of life. First defined in Frankl, V.E. (1949). *Der unbedingte Mensch*. Vienna: Franz Deuticke.

putting a heroic, positive model into the world, something good which propagates itself.

As the group moves into a deeper exploration, it is necessary to consider the quantity of values as well as their quality. For we know that every instance of despair has an act of idolizing as its ultimate basis; *behind every despair lies an idol.* It is dangerous to cling to a single value in life and to place it at the peak of a pyramid of values; the peak breaks off all too easily and leaves behind a pile of ruins.

It is psychologically healthier to have a personal value system which has many values and various equally important life areas. Should the value of life be challenged to its core, it is helpful to use an image we have regarding depression. We can equate some kinds of depressions to dark clouds in the sky, which we should just patiently let pass over because we are sure that the sun is still shining above them. In a similar way, we can be sure that life's horizon of meaning and values never disappears, not even when we temporarily do not see it.

The caption "depression" leads into the discussion of serious questions of life, like the questions of *fate, guilt, suffering* and *death*. Concerning the accidents of fate to which we are more or less exposed, Frankl's comment is an important discovery that "we are not what is asking the question, rather we are answering it." Participants at this stage learn to cease to rail against their unalterable fate and instead learn to explore the possibilities still open to them in each case in order to respond to the challenges of fate. They thus experience themselves at least as codeterminers of their destiny and not merely as its helpless victims.

Some of the group members may have already realized in their own lives how the meaning of guilt and suffering so very often lies in experiencing the pain of growing into better forms of the self. The question of whether death does not make life meaningless has passed sometime through everyone's lips. It is therefore of great prophylactic importance to carefully present the logotherapeutic argument that, on the contrary, it is the fact of death which makes life meaningful. For it is death which forces us to act here and now, because there is nothing that can be put off indefinitely. The image of the full granary of the past, in which the harvest of our lives remains protected in safekeeping, supports our thinking, even if our view of the stubble fields after harvesting at the end of our life frightens us.

During such serious reflections, it is unavoidable that we move sooner or later to the *area of religion*. Of course, the logotherapeutic meditation group should never be misused to represent just one specific religious opinion, or to consider one religion as better than another. Logotherapy is a form of psychotherapy, but as such it also cannot evade the pressing concerns of its patients. In this context it is helpful to mention the view of the various religions which function like the various languages of mankind: None is superior to any others, and we can approach the truth with each language. Since it is possible that there are also convicted atheists in the meditation group, it is meaningful to pass on Frankl's definition of God as "the partner of our most intimate conversations." This definition is acceptable to people of every worldview: Those who believe in God, pray; those who do not believe in God, talk to themselves or with their own conscience.

At the conclusion of the meditation group, it is noted that a healthy noödynamic—a healthy tension between "being" and "ought"—is irrevocably necessary and that we should not try to avoid it. A life without ups and downs is an empty life, and a life which serves only to satisfy one's own needs is a life devoid of meaning. Participants may not expect of their lives that it will always be pleasant and comfortable, but they do have a right to expect that it will always and everywhere have meaningful possibilities; whether they see and fulfill these possibilities of meaning depends on them and them alone.

The third stage of our logotherapeutic procedure culminates with the strong conviction that life must be and can be mastered, and that there are no situations for which there is not also some inner attitude that is suitable to manage it. Participants learned at the first stage to master their weaknesses, at the second stage to build up their strengths, and now at the third stage they learned to accept and to affirm life independently of weaknesses and strengths, ups and downs. With a wealth of philosophical concepts of logotherapy, which the group members can combine any way they like with their own worldview, they have gained an inner stability that will not be abandoned even in times of crisis.

At this point, little remains to be done. It is more or less only a symbolic act, but an important, demonstrative line drawing an end to the patients' histories of illness; they now enter into *self-responsibility*. Human society values certain symbols which indicate rites of passage; for example, the age when a person is no longer a minor, graduation diplomas, wedding announcements. A similar purpose is fulfilled by the short individual sessions which I conduct at the *fourth stage* with participants who are graduating into life. These are conversations which should make it clear to such individuals that the therapist-patient relationship has been set aside, because they are no longer patients.

In order to confer a special emphasis to the "once-and-for-all cure," I purposely do not offer any advice at all at the fourth stage; I become an equal partner in the conversation and chat about this or that without the slightest intention of exercising influence on their lives. These conversations may seem superfluous at first glance, but I am convinced that they are indirectly very important; they let former patients understand that henceforth the full responsibility for their actions and deeds is, as a matter of fact, delegated to them, and that the therapist will in no way make their decisions easier. It is the clear and unmistakable knowledge of being psychologically healthy again, but also of being alone responsible for one's life. These two considerations, which belong indissolubly together, should put an end to any next relapse. These individuals can free themselves completely of any dependence on therapy. But only if they actually experience the therapist not taking care of them at all and not being willing to again pull pat solutions out of the drawer for them, although the therapist is still ready to stay in contact with them as a person and friend.

Until the end of the third stage (including participation in both of the groups), I leave open the possibility of additional sessions of individual therapy for any problems which happen to arise. But I do not do this at the fourth stage. Either the patient is cured, or we have to start all over again, because something has gone wrong. But then the question comes up of whether the illness is not resistant to therapy and whether it would be better to work on making the patient's life worthy of living with and in spite of any illness, something which is sometimes also considered.

Regardless, at the fourth stage I conduct superficial, friendly conversations about interesting daily topics with the clear accentuation of two healthy and rational persons just talking together. In this way I overcome the memory of the style of the individual sessions of the first stage, which was characterized by the helplessness and partial incapacity of the individual and by the "higher position" of the therapist as a person consulted for help. The person to be released should not get the idea of running back to the counselor whenever a little problem arises, and he must therefore get to know him or her as someone who is not always only understanding, attentive and ready to help. As remarkable as it sounds, the therapist should not signal the same helpfulness at the end of the therapy as it was at the beginning, if the client is to be prevented from leaving in a state of dependence. The process of "cutting the umbilical cord" can only be initiated by the therapist acting in an atypical manner, which plays an essential role in the question of how permanent the effect of therapy will be.

This does not mean that therapists should behave in a rejecting or offensive manner but like good parents allow their grown children be independent—they are careful not to tell them what to do, thus refraining from helping them too much with their everyday problems. In this way, logotherapists let individuals leave when they reach the fourth stage; such counselors do not call after them, causing them to turn around and come back. And if some should turn around with some doubts still in their hearts, then the only thing which may be said to them is something that equally applies to all of us, namely that they should listen to the voice of their own minds and follow their own conscience.

As far as one can judge, the cured individuals now live "selflessly", that is, without continuously brooding about themselves and their situations. They live "happily" insofar as they live meaningfully, and they live "their" lives without help or therapeutic intervention from outside. Only when these individuals have really become clear about that have they truly entered the spiritual level of maturity of self-responsibility and can be handed over without hesitation to life. Parting after the fourth stage is simple and without complication. The paths of two persons have touched each other for awhile; now they split apart and both move further on, trusting that their encounter has not been without significance.

Perhaps the whole program for the reduction of the danger of relapses in psychotherapy, which I have just very briefly presented, may seem a little arbitrary, as if it could just as well be composed of other levels. But almost a decade of logotherapeutic research stands behind it. Whoever has explored as I have the wealth and multidimensionality of this form of psychotherapy, must come to the conclusion, that its deepest secret and its greatest blessing is present in the concept of *self-transcendence* and in its *openness to the possibilities of spiritual growth*. Logotherapy was never a method for merely treating symptoms. It does not take its patients back into the dark, unconscious past, but it does lead them further into a bright, clearly conscious future. And in order to be able to take individuals into this future, we need therapeutic levels that build on each other like those I have sketched. They can, of course, be modified, but fundamentally they must run along the tracks of strengthening self-transcendence and the promotion of spiritual growth.

A symbol can illustrate more vividly what in scientific terms can only be expressed much too dispassionately. Let us assume that those who need psychotherapeutic treatment are defined as those who have stumbled and fallen over the obstacles and rough times of their lives; they cannot get up again on their own.

At the first stage of the logotherapeutic program, they will be brought to their feet and provided with crutches to which they can cling. These crutches are methods such as paradoxical intention, dereflection, attitude modulation and all other procedures including those from other types of therapy, which can be combined to overcome the actual crisis. After completion of psychotherapeutic treatment, those who are on crutches risk the first fearful steps alone. But they still walk slowly and hobble, their heads down, tensely watching each step. The fear of falling again still plagues them

10. Admssion Into Self-Responsibility: Reducing the Relapse Rate

and makes them lean heavily on their crutches. It makes their legs tremble and unsteady. With their heads down, the patients see nothing of their surroundings; they grope blindly forward, happy even just to get moving.

This is the point where many therapies stop; the clients can walk again, and the rest is assumed to be a matter of practice. However, it is premature to release them at this time; the hyperreflection about the crises suffered, the present instability and the constriction of their fields of view, which blocks their perceptions of future goals could quickly produce a sudden relapse. In the dereflection group of the second stage, participants first learn to raise their heads and to stop tensely watching their own steps. They learn to walk trustfully with their crutches, while seeing the surrounding world. Dereflection is always like *gently lifting the chin* of convalescents, upon which they stop looking down at the floor and glance into the distance, upon which their spiritual horizon is also broadened and they become aware of the meaningful tasks and precious values of life. At the second stage, they still walk with crutches, but they do so resolutely and standing straight. They can look around at the world and fix their eyes upon their personal, positive goals.

What could continue to cause a relapse is the possibility of stumbling over the unevenness of the ground, where unsteady feet can get caught, caused by new problems coming up that cause a stumble. Therefore, individuals must learn at the third level—in the logotherapeutic meditation group—how to walk in *every* kind of terrain. Metaphorically speaking, they learn how to climb over rocks and to keep their balance on ice; they learn how to bridge swamps and make their way through the thorns. Meditations from the logotherapeutic treasury show them scenarios of life with which they will someday be confronted. And they find attitudes towards these situations that make it possible for spiritual growth in spite of them. Whatever problems they will face, whether emotional frustration or bodily sickness, whether an external problem or an inner fear of death, such individuals will have a concrete idea at hand which can be used like a rope to pull themselves up when their knees begin to wobble or an attack of dizziness becomes overwhelming. After the third stage, participants can not only walk with crutches, they can not only walk with their heads raised, now they can go *everywhere*, in any direction they may choose, on any street which destiny may lead them to.

The time has come, on the basis of a newly gained stability and above all in recognition of the self-responsibility which has been acquired, to send each individual on the way without any supporting devices. At the fourth stage, a level of spiritual maturity is attained which allows them to ceremoniously throw the crutches in the corner and to walk firmly on both feet on a path that is taken purposefully and willingly, a path on which they will stay to the end, even when great shadows fall upon it. And if the path should lead into the darkness of night, or should it someday become impassable, the memory of the logotherapeutic insights will still reveal a gleam of hope on the horizon, which may save them from falling into the abyss of despair.

Table 1 summarizes the most important characteristics of this program for the reduction of the relapse rate in psychotherapy.

Of course, I am aware that the program described represents the ideal case. The unique and individual nature of each individual, with which we are concerned, involves the possibility that therapy may fail. We are neither psychological mechanics, nor are we dealing with automated mechanisms that can be broken down into their components and then put back together again. But even when we know that we will occasionally fail in our efforts, we still have the obligation to set the highest possible therapeutic goals. What we are concerned with is also the highest known earthly value: human existence.

Whoever really wants to cure, must want to cure once and for all. And whoever really loves his or her patients, must let them finally enter into self-responsibility.

Stage	Session type	Concept	Main consideration	Logotherapeutic contribution	Mobilizing the human capacity for	Symbol of individual steps
First	Individual	Problem solving and symptom reduction	In the negative (problem) and in the positive (solution)	Specific logotherapeutic techniques (paradoxical intention, attitude modulation) and combined methods to re-establish freedom of will	Self-detachment	Is barely able to walk with crutches
Second	Group	Dereflection group (for general dereflection)	Only in the positive (stipulation)	Logotherapy's theory of the person, defining a will to meaning (noëtic dimension)	Self-transcendence	No longer intensely watches each step, but rather looks up from the floor and sees the environment
Third	Group	Logotherapeutic meditation group (for prophylaxis)	In the negative (blows of fate) and in the positive (coping)	Philosophical principles of logotherapy, defining life to have meaning under all circumstances	Transforming suffering into a meaningful achievement	Learns how to walk in every kind of field, regardless of difficulty
Fourth	Individual	Release and admission into self-responsibility	Only in the positive (setting aside the therapist-patient relationship)	Logotherapy's fundamental concern, raising the spiritual level of the human being	Comprehending freedom as self-responsibility	Puts crutches aside and enters the world as a healthy person

Table 1: A four-stage logotherapeutic program for the reduction of the relapse rate in psychotherapy

"How free am I?"
Man asks his Creator.

"I cannot discard
my body,
I cannot deny
my ancestry,
I cannot flee from
my environment,
I cannot escape from
my time."

"You are not free
from your conditions".
He replies,
"but you are free
to choose an attitude
to your conditions.

And that is more
than I ever granted."

Elisabeth Lukas

CHAPTER 11

Reflections on our Future (2014)

After more than seven decades of experience in life, I dare say that life is full of surprises. But not only good ones, I must admit. Sometimes, life surprises us with unexpected blows of fate and rough provocations. On the other hand, we can give life the credit it deserves, for it also surprises us with fascinating offers and totally unexpected gifts.

The fact that I stand here today is one of these gifts. I have given lectures, seminars, workshops, etc. at 53 universities, but never at the University of Moscow. My books have been published in 17 languages, but none of them in Russian. That the fame of my humble work in the area of logotherapy has reached Russia is truly a big surprise life granted me.

If I may, I would like to add the following to the subject of life's surprises: It is important to remain receptive and alert for them well into old age. It is known that fear of the new and the unusual is one sign of a neurotic existence. What we are used to, the familiar and the mundane, are markers of security that, in fact, never exist. We are able to navigate the familiar, what we are used to and think we know, and thus believe we are able to master life. However, the more we tend to trust that we can manage the known, the more shocking are experiences of abrupt changes

---

This address was delivered by Elisabeth Lukas on May 18, 2014 at the Billrothhaus of the Vienna Medical Society at the ceremony to confer an honorary professorship on her during the 2014 "The Future of Logotherapy II" Congress in Vienna, organized by the Viktor Frankl Institute Vienna.

and new situations. To stay open to the changes of time, which also requires letting go and changing direction, will provide more flexibility to react to the surprises of life when they hit us in the face.

One of the many supportive strategies of logotherapy is preventive: to train us not to freeze or to feel completely overwhelmed when faced with life's surprises, but to tackle them with a degree of serenity. How did I reach this conclusion? Frankl's philosophy enters so intensely into the full spectrum of human existence that the more we penetrate into it, the more we start to engage with all possible surprises of life. In our realm of thought, we already start to move along paths for which the future alone can build.

If, for example, we study Frankl's assertions about the tragic triad, we definitely encounter our own suffering, our own guilt, our own death so that, in our imagination, there is hardly a rift between what we have suffered and what we are still to suffer. Or, if we study the Franklian triad of values, we experience a happy balance between creative accomplishments, the bliss of love, the pride of courage; again, the gap between what was and what is yet to come shrinks. "Everything we see is harvest, even if it is still in the fields, or maybe already stored in the barn." This is one of Frankl's most well-known sayings. Logotherapy is indeed able to equip us for the process of a continuous harvest, come what may; to enable us to deal with pain as well as to foster the boundless estimation of grace.

At my age, of course, I am well aware of the passing nature of all worldly splendors; I know that possessions, power, prestige, and honor are extremely relative and quickly go up in smoke. But this celebration is very special for me because it is tied to people that mean a lot to me. To be precise, I must first thank my writings and second, my students, for the honor of being here. Without my writings and without my loyal and talented former students, such as Professor Batthyány, nobody in Moscow would ever have noticed me. But to whom do I owe my writings, and to whom do I owe my students?

I owe my literary activity to Prof. Frankl. In 1978, he urged me to write a book about my experiences of the practical applications of logotherapy. Personally, I would not have had the confidence to write the book, but my

11. Reflections on our Future

first work emerged due to his insistence and literally because of my esteem for him. The ice was broken....

How did I get my wonderful students? These I owe to my husband, who in 1985 took the initiative to smooth the difficult path for the foundation of our Institute of Logotherapy in southern Germany, in Fürstenfeldbruck near Munich. I did not have the confidence to head a scientific institute with an outpatient psychotherapy clinic, but he had faith in me, and so a place of training was established, in cooperation, where over the years more than a thousand experts graduated in logotherapy.

This is why I dedicate this personal tribute to Professor Frankl and to my husband. They both have contributed decisively to my entire personal evolution. Both were like beacons in a stormy sea for me, making sure that my boat of life did not capsize, sink, or get lost somewhere in the dark.

I regret that my husband is now in the hospital and cannot be with us. But I feel him close in thought and as if he were on my side as he has always been. I just want to share with you one of his innumerable small gestures: When I lectured in the United States or Canada, my husband was given the rare opportunity to fly an aircraft. He held an American pilot's license and fuel was much more affordable in the U.S. than in Germany. But he, the passionate pilot, remained by my side in the auditorium.

Professor Frankl wrote famous essays on spiritual "being with" (*Bei Sein*), "to be with the things that interest us" (*Bei den Dingen unseres Interesses Sein*), "being with the people we love" (*Bei den Menschen unserer Liebe Sein*) a "being with," which certainly longs for a physical expression, but does not depend on physical presence per se, so I can well imagine that he is right now present among us.

Based on the understanding of the importance of encouragement at the right time, I personally would like to encourage the officials of the University of Moscow not to be irritated by any obstacles or psychological countercurrents and to continue the teaching task that has been started to integrate Frankl's thought into their curriculum. It will be of much benefit to them and to their students.

I guess I am not mistaken when I say that there have been many changes in Russia in recent decades. People are moving on from a troubled past. In Central Europe, too, there have been massive changes. The Greek phrase "pánta rei" (πάντα ρει, everything is in flow) holds a deep truth. Frankl's phrase "every age has its neuroses and every age needs its therapy" is also very true. Throughout my life alone, I have been able to observe a great variety of stages this country has gone through. I would like to briefly describe, what I have experienced, even though I can only refer to the situation in my own country:

- First, there was poverty after World War II. I was only a child and we had—like most—barely enough to live. There were no toys, no winter heating, etc. I remember my grandfather crossing Vienna with a backpack to reach the potato fields north of the Danube River because of a rumor that there were potatoes for sale there. When he came back at night, tired and with an empty backpack because he had gone too late, I heard my mother cry. And yet, I experienced that part of my life with a profound sense of security. We were together; everybody helped each other, and values still existed.

- Then came the growing prosperity of the 1950s, and with it, great joy. I have never again perceived so much joy in my social circles. I was in high school and I was happy. One could buy a book, afford a new dress, and… dear God!… get a bicycle. It was like intoxication and it ended like one.

- The economic miracle (*Wirtschaftswunder*) of the 1960s overwhelmed us and let all traditional values crumble. A wave of sexual indulgence flooded us, authorities were toppled, and people were beside themselves. Suddenly everyone wanted to be his or her "true self," no matter at whose expense. All this happened while I was attended the university and I was pulled in by the trends of this rebellious period. If I had not met Viktor Frankl, who knows what psychological labyrinth I would have lost myself in?

- Economic well-being expanded and joy faded away. A new generation grew up in the late 1970s: the "no-future generation" as they called themselves sarcastically. Their label was "*Null Bock auf Nichts*" (I can't be bothered about anything). Since I was already familiar with logotherapy, I recognized the symptoms of the existential vacuum, which took hold of people and swallowed them alive. There were cars and housing for all, there was enough work, there were all kinds of liberties people could wish for, there were opportunities for adventurous travel, and yet… increases in depression, suicide, freaky young people, drug addicts, and crimes of meaningless violence and destruction.

By this time, I was working as a psychologist; through my patients I got to know unnecessary self-inflicted suffering and pain that affected them and those around them, a result of their own discontent, displeasure, boredom, indifference, and selfishness. From the saying: "primum vivere, deinde philosophari" (first food, then philosophy) I learned: After too much food, there is no more morality. Frankl had already prophetically predicted, even before World War II when there was no idea of luxury and excessive pleasures, that it is not good for the psyche of man when he is too well off outwardly and materialistically.

- Progress moved on worldwide, and at a dizzying pace. With technology and globalization, a new era dawned. Suddenly, everything was connected via networks and the world's problems began rattling the prosperity of the pampered nations.

The end of the millennium brought the realization that resources were starting to dwindle. Work and money started to become scarce. But as little as many people in my country had appreciated their prosperity, just as little were they ready to do without it. Their mentality began to develop into the direction of our current society. People work hard to maintain a high standard of living, but stress charges a high price. Mobbing, envy, competitive infighting, panic attacks, physical exhaustion, burnout, and symptoms of strain are psychological issues of the day. To this, add the addiction to drifting off in front of the television screen or computer monitor, which is allowed to progressively absorb the soul of its viewer. Economic crises, energy crises, and crises in the family are common today.

Amidst all this, there is an immense yearning for tranquility, peace, and well-being, for a simple life instead of constant struggles in the workplace, and in the complicated relationships of human interaction as we see them all around us. I am past the stress now. I no longer work. I have been living in a happy marriage for 44 years, and have a good relationship with our children. But I feel a great degree of compassion for the younger generations.

The spiritual question is present in each of these stages. It raises its head in poverty and wealth alike, in need and in abundance. If the development of these processes is carefully considered, we can see a trend that Frankl had already sensed for some time and explained with the increasing loss of tradition and instinct in mankind: In our digital age we are left alone more and more in our search for answers to our spiritual questions.

It has become disturbingly difficult to form an opinion that makes sense. Does it make sense to grow genetically modified wheat? Does it make sense to entrust children to life partners of the same gender? Does it make sense to give loans to foreign companies? Does it make sense to enter personal information on the Internet? Every day, we are presented with an endless set of questions, which no one can answer objectively or reasonably, because the arguments for and against appear to be in balance.

The media are the opinion makers. Depending on economic, political, or religious positions, they bombard the individual with selective pseudo-arguments for which a person has barely any defenses. Each television ad tells of a hidden "meaning" of the actions of its protagonists; great strength of character—or, even better, continence—is required, in order to escape these subtle manipulations.

It is possible that this situation varies in Russia or in other continents. However, there, too, the stage is set more and more by the gripping attempt of each individual to find meaning in life in light of its manifold contradictions and influences and thus to shape one's own actions in a

11. Reflections on our Future

meaningful way. According to psychological studies, we are currently living in a renaissance of the question of meaning because meaning has become so doubtful, almost fragile.

So what can Viktor Frankl offer us, whose teachings have been at the foundation of this phenomenon of meaning for almost a hundred years, in the light of these extreme transformations of the postmodern era? As you can see, I am reversing the theme of the conference a little bit. I am not worried about the "future of logotherapy." Logotherapy will constantly gain in importance, but the future itself gives reason for worry. Therefore, I would like to pursue the question: What perspectives of logotherapy prepare us for the future? In the building of Frankl's teaching, there are profound aspects of hope that are highly relevant. Let me mention four of them because they appear particularly important to me.

First, the aspect of *conscience*—the human organ of meaning: Although terribly slow to develop, conscience is being refined with the progress of culture. We are beings with such short lifespans that it is difficult to see the progress. But Frankl, with his broad vision, observed that, beyond the pathologies of each respective Zeitgeist, there are and have been throughout history mutations of sentiment on a grand scale that push us in a positive direction. He made it evident with the example of slavery, which was once considered legal but is now proscribed worldwide. Today, similar streams of thought and opinion emerge around the globe, especially among the young. Supported by the means of modern communication, making everything infinitely more transparent than before, more and more nations rise against dictatorship, corruption, terror, and tyranny. Unfortunately, these mass protests rarely occur without the employment of arms, which is certainly not consistent with a collective revolution of awareness. Regardless, a glimmer of hope is emerging on the horizon: Brutal tyrants are finding it increasingly hard to gag their subjects and rob them because the resistance and self-confidence of nations grow, enabling them to struggle for freedom, self-determination, and the safeguard of their human rights.

Joseph Fabry, a longtime friend of Frankl, once commented on a discussion in which Frankl described conscience not only as the most intimate pathfinder of the individual but also as a tool of human evolution. Frankl believed—and I quote,

> In a society that universally accepted cannibalism, only a person with an exceedingly refined conscience would have been able to contradict the environment in which he was brought up. When that person's conscience contradicted cannibalism, he became a revolutionary. He may have been killed, but he was able to awaken the conscience of others. This is the way human progress takes place.[1]

This is an excellent example, because it does not imply that he, who was not a cannibal, attacked or exterminated his partners, who still were. The "rebel" in Frankl's picture is a pacifist; he refuses to harm human dignity and, if necessary, abides by the consequences. Today, if the increase of protests of nations against prevailing injustices, against the impoverishment of many and the enrichment beyond measure of a few would go hand in hand with the amazing accomplishments of peaceful resistance by conviction, indeed a progress of humaneness would be within reach.

The second aspect of hope I am detecting is the *widespread longing for a break* from the daily turmoil. Twenty years ago, the slogan "to be ripe for the island" produced a smile, but also a remarkable echo. Since then, the dream of time off, if at all affordable, is alive in the minds of many people, as long as one can afford it. Not always is the urge to escape the impetus for it.

A feeling of wanting to leave the infamous rat race has emerged, that there should be an opportunity to escape the constant sensory overload and to live a simpler life with more awareness and authenticity. Although this is frequently not feasible, a strong vision forms in that regard in the hearts of many people, which could become increasingly more fertile in its intensity.

Viktor Frankl once argued on a radio show that

> Man should learn again to go into the desert for a while, for a weekend perhaps—and there are deserts nearby, they are

---

[1] Cited in Fabry, J. (2013). *The pursuit of meaning.* Charlottesville: Purpose Research, p. 69.

11. Reflections on our Future

everywhere; whether a hike to a mountain hut, or a secluded bay on a shore. There, at least, one can finish thinking one's own thoughts....

Frankl, who already in his youth was identified as a "thinker who thinks things through" (*Zu Ende Denker*).

Yes, our thoughts! Consider this: There are not only two kinds of feelings—the purely basic feelings of hunger, fear, anger, greed, etc., and the specifically human feelings of sense of value, friendship, enthusiasm, artistic or scientific fascination, etc., as described by Frankl in his book: *Der unbewusste Gott (The unconscious God)*.[1]

There are also two modes of thinking: on the one side, intelligence, logic, memory, etc., and on the other the specifically human level of wisdom, understanding, insight, and acceptance. The former is based on cortical performance; the latter goes beyond mere physiology, as it involves the human spirit.

Frankl was right, of course: Only in silence, in a withdrawal of stimulation, that is, in our personal "desert," are we able to "think through" something in peace, to feel what we really want or must do, to clearly see what "makes sense just now," to discern what should receive our wholehearted "Yes." However, most people are no longer used to this way of thinking.

I would like to give you a simple example. I wrote my first 10 books on my typewriter. This was tiring, because every page had to be typed several times, from draft to final text. As it was difficult to correct mistakes on the typewriter, it was necessary to develop the ability to formulate entire paragraphs in my head and to write them down, print-ready, in one pass.

The following principle prevailed: "think first, then act"—in my example: Think through a phrase first and then write it down. When computers arrived, it became incomparably more convenient, and no one can do without word processing nowadays. But the principle changed. Because you can correct, change, delete, and conceptualize again, today the principle

---

[1] The English translation of this book has been revised and republished as Frankl, V. E. (2000). *Man's search for ultimate meaning*. Cambridge: Perseus.

is: "act first—then think"; in this example, write a half-baked phrase and then correct or delete it. When writing a book, this may not be that serious, but in life, "act first—then think" is not at all a principle I recommend because a poor thought process can no longer be corrected and could easily become a boomerang.

In life, today's generation, too, should stick to, or rather return to "think first—then act" and this is much easier if there is a general habit of making excursions into the private desert, where in silence we can think things through, where we encounter our true inner selves, where we can hear the spiritual calling of the hour. This regenerative step into the desert, however, requires a sacrifice: self-restraint and humility.

Those who fill their free time with events and entertainment, shopping, surfing, talking on the phone, and other pastimes will have the same experience as those who stuff their homes with things they do not need; they drown in the clutter. Clearing things out, slowing down, and a new frugality are the liberating elements, which place the innermost longings of the human being, at least in our Western society—that is, longings completely different from those our constant advertising promises to fulfill—within our reach. Let us hope for a new culture of reflection; it could help to change the face of the Earth for the better.

The computer leads us to the third aspect of hope: With the advent of technology, *mankind has created a "third brain,"* despite all prophecies of doom from the turmoil of our time. In addition to its archaic brainstem, with its automatic and homeostatic regulation of performance, and its amazingly integrative associative layer, the neocortex, *Homo sapiens* now also has powerful computers available, capable of delivering information extracted from huge data files almost instantly, which human analyzing and research alone could never have been able to produce. Aside from this, the information provided by the computer is not affected by emotions and assumptions, as is the case in the process of human thought.

Of course, everything can be abused, as bad experiences with the Internet have shown. How wise was Frankl, when he stated that things never depend on a given technology but on the spirit in which they are

11. Reflections on our Future

handled. But apart from any abuse, the "third brain" opens opportunities we never guessed at to access the real secrets of being, which surround and include us, and to get to know and to better understand reality. Anyone who has worked therapeutically with those seeking advice knows how much depends on an adequate assessment of reality. Not only does misjudgment of reality dramatically impair the lives of psychotically ill patients; patients with psychological and emotional disturbances also suffer from unrealistic fears and imaginary drowning of the self.

Even individuals that can be considered psychologically healthy sometimes act against their realistic situations, by getting into debt that they cannot afford, eating foods that are harmful, or hastily agreeing to do things they cannot face. Failure to accept reality is a process of self-punishment, which usually has bad consequences, both in big and in small things. Historians, for example, have demonstrated that both World Wars of the previous century started by a flawed assessment of reality—not just among those in charge inside the political machinery, but also among the broad population. The more crystallized that ideologies become, the more they slip away from reality.

This "third brain" can, if used properly, help to assess reality correctly. With its help, a vehicle has been landed on Mars—just to mention one detail among millions. To achieve such a success, immense precision and the analysis of many physical relations are necessary. The slightest error, for example in the calculation of the trajectory, might have ruined the whole project. To be sure, computers cannot determine whether it makes any sense at all to land on Mars. But when we, humans beings, believe something makes sense, computers might be able to inform us whether it is possible and how we can accomplish it.

We started with the problem that, due to the complexity of our time, it has become more difficult to distinguish between what makes sense and what does not. But nobody can take this task of discernment from us; it remains the responsibility par excellence of the human being.

However, faced with these difficulties, more and more sophisticated machines are able to provide detailed information for the feasibility of our plans, for the prediction of the consequences of our actions, for the realistic effects of grave interventions in nature, and so on. They can be placed at the service of the search for—and the discovery of—meaning, as they filter out illusions and join ideals with feasibility.

The condition is that they are put to service, that is, they serve, and that human beings control them and not the other way around. This needs to be worked on and I believe it is the biggest task for today's generation: To turn computers on *and off*, to use them for meaning-oriented purposes without succumbing to them and to their seductions. If the new generation succeeds, we will be able to achieve tremendous results for the future with the help of our "third brain."

I still want to address a fourth hopeful aspect, the controversial topic of *globalization*, which stirs the minds and certainly cannot be turned back. To the contrary, everything in this world starts to mix and everything that happens has effects on everything else. Single nations can no longer "cook their own soup"; other nations throw alien ingredients into their pot, whether they like it or not. We can complain about it, rage against it, but we know from psychotherapy that counterpositions per se are not constructive.

Positive results can be found in a creative acceptance; in this case, an acceptance of a world that is worth being lived in. Frankl's saying that "the world is not healthy, but it can be healed," is still valid, especially today.

What, then, could contribute to healing in this age of unstoppable and unavoidable moving closer together?

Let's think about this: Why is there so much friction between neighbors near and far? The answer: because we are so different. Different races, different world views, different parties, different desires and worries, different capacities, different age-old adjustments to different environments… endless differences.… How, then, can we possibly understand each other?

Nevertheless, we share in a great—a splendid—common denominator, and we truly owe it to Viktor Frankl. We do not just have a clue, but the weight of his decisive words: *Each human being of every nation is a spiritual, noëtic person. This is the only fundamental bond between us all.* This is what unites us: the spiritual dimension and, with it, freedom, responsibility, creative potential, and boundless and inalienable personal dignity.

Although it sounds astonishing, it is just this phenomenon of globalization that might become helpful when we consider our common ground. From the understanding that our well-being and suffering are united, that nobody can escape looming disasters, such as climate threats, and that in the future we will either all be well or miserable, there is a chance for a single credo to arise in unison, roughly equivalent to what Frankl had already claimed decades ago, *a monanthropism*: faith in our common humanity, of which we are all part—a faith that would be able to bridge all the differences, which today confuse us so desperately.

As one of the first students of Frankl, allow me to say, then, what Frankl would most likely have offered to the human being on the path of search for meaning at the beginning of the 21st century. I think he would say: "Get up! Rise against the permanent causation of suffering that surrounds you; open your subtle sense for true values and fight for tolerance and mutual respect—but renounce counteraggression and any other angry fighting.

Frankl taught us that bad means desecrate the best cause. In his forcefully moving play *Synchronization in Buchenwald*, Frankl left us a calling: "We shall not go on forever repaying hate with hate, injustice with injustice, force with force! The chain, Paul—the chain, that's it—it must be broken!"[1] It is a heritage that could not be more convincing.

Frankl might continue like this: "Be frugal. Do not get lured by the siren calls of consumerism and take a little break in your personal desert. Listen to the voice of transcendence!" He advised us, in a time when the Ten Commandments seem to lose their validity, to observe the 10,000 rules hiding in the 10,000 situations in our complicated lives.

But, how can anyone perceive 10,000 rules? It is simple. They manifest themselves to us in silence, piece by piece… not as strict commands from "above," but as loving whispers of the truest friend we have: our conscience.

---

1 Spoken by "Franz" in the unpublished English translation of Frankl, V. E. (1945). *Synchronization in Buchenwald* (Joseph Fabry, trans.), p. 35.

Frankl probably would continue by saying:

> Meanwhile, you have accumulated an amazing technical repertoire, which provides you with enormous opportunities, but be careful with it! Any technological feature needs to be controlled by something metatechnical, so as not to turn against its own inventors.

Frankl elucidated, based on psychotherapeutic techniques, that even art and wisdom are not enough if they are not paired with the human aspect—that human aspect that gives technology its adequate place and sets its limits.

Frankl might add:

> Don't ever forget, you are the being who always decides. You decide what you will be in the next moment. You, due to your spiritual faculties, are the active collaborator of your fate. United in one mankind, you are the active contributor to human history.
>
> With your actions, you are writing in a book of history from which nothing can be erased, not the glorious and not the awful, but which still has an unknown number of pages, white, blank pages, which at the end will testify on your behalf. Turn this into a communal epic worthy of you.

I remember an anecdote Frankl used to tell about some students who were not talking to each other, until the day their bus got stuck in the mud. Suddenly, they were working shoulder to shoulder to free the bus, and any disagreements between them vanished. Frankl emphasized that there was nothing as placating as a common meaningful task. Therefore, he would probably close with these words:

> Take these children as an example! There are enough treasures in the world that can be released from the mud with joined forces. Work with confidence, shoulder to shoulder, each person with his or her own talents, so that the "tragic optimism" that I have upheld all *my* life, will in *your* lives gradually turn to a "justified optimism."

I cannot express it more beautifully than did Viktor Frankl; let us thank him for his inspiration and example.

11. Reflections on our Future

Don't laugh about
the "sane world"—
it has a chance
as long as it exists
at least in our longing.

> Don't ridicule
> the "sane world"—
> it remains accessible
> as long as it exists
> at least in our language.

>> Don't gamble away
>> the "sane world"—
>> it still can become reality
>> as long as we don't abandon it
>> in our thoughts.

>> Elisabeth Lukas

Lightning Source UK Ltd.
Milton Keynes UK
UKHW020636230222
399120UK00009B/539